G000138019

Hands

A Clinical Companion

Steps to confidence in musculoskeletal diagnosis

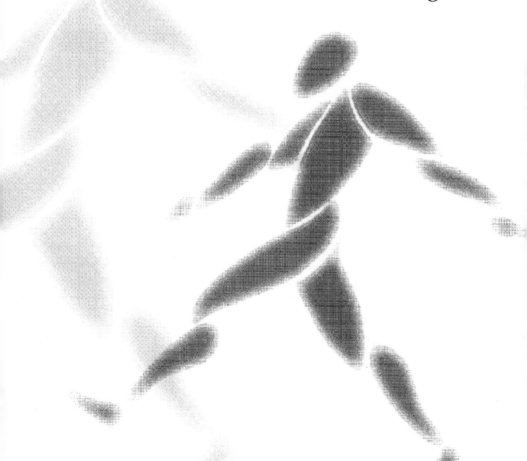

Simon Browning DO Cert Ed

tfm Publishing Limited
Castle Hill Barns
Harley
Nr Shrewsbury
SY5 6LX
UK

Tel: +44 (0)1952 510061; Fax: +44 (0)1952 510192
E-mail: nikki@tfmpublishing.co.uk; Web site: www.tfmpublishing.co.uk

Design and layout: Nikki Bramhill
Illustrators: Simon Browning
                       Marcus Bernini

Printed by Cromwell Press Ltd, Aintree Avenue, White Horse Business Park, Trowbridge, Wiltshire, BA14 0XB, UK

Tel: +44 (0)1225 711400; Fax: +44 (0)1225 711429

Contents

SECTION III

Foreword

I have been working in private practice as an osteopath for over twenty-five years and have recently returned to the teaching environment. Over the years, it has become apparent to me that a practical clinical handbook that can be used as an aide-memoir will assist both the senior student and experienced practitioner who are keen to embrace the concept of continued professional development.

This handbook draws together into one place information from a range of medical, orthopaedic and anatomical textbooks. By design it provides only the basic information, enough for the busy practitioner in the clinic and sufficient to encourage further reading if gaps in personal knowledge are identified.

The handbook is divided into three sections. Section one reviews the initial consultation process from the case history, red flag issues to the physical assessment of the patient. Section two concentrates on specific joints and areas in the body reviewing in turn the anatomy, causes of symptoms, the normal physical findings and special tests. Section three, although addressing gait and neurological assessments, focuses on the causes of other symptoms with which a patient may present, including multiple joint pain, abdominal pain, chest pain and headaches.

This handbook is NOT designed to give:-

   ♦   a detailed description of every cause of every symptom possible;
   ♦   all the specific signs and symptoms of common musculoskeletal problems;
   ♦   the full range of special tests that can be used to determine tissue causing symptoms.

.... as this information is readily available in specialist medical texts.

Books, even medical texts, are a personal choice and you will gain much from them if they are presented in a way you find easy to read. Although I will not recommend specific textbooks to add to your clinical library, I suggest that you have books that cover the following subject areas:-

♦ anatomy;
♦ clinical examination;
♦ medicine;
♦ neurology;
♦ orthopaedic assessment;
♦ orthopaedics;
♦ rheumatology.

Many of these standard medical texts paint a clinical picture that is black and white with no shades of grey. It is, consequently, essential to remember to keep an open mind, a flexible outlook and a willingness to embrace the unexpected or improbable when examining or treating patients. With experience you notice that patients:-

♦ do not necessarily have the classic signs and symptoms associated with a specific condition;
♦ frequently report symptoms differently, depending on how the question was asked;
♦ often tell the practitioner what they think s/he wants to hear;
♦ have one presenting complaint that encompasses several problems.

Acknowledgements

I would like to thank my wife Jill for her patience, perseverance and proof-reading. I would also like to thank my colleagues and students at the London School of Osteopathy for their comments, suggestions and corrections. Finally, I am indebted to Carol West, a qualified osteopath with experience in publishing, who proof-read the entire book with a very critical eye.

Simon Browning
January 2004

Chapter 1

Case history

Listen to the patient, he is telling you the diagnosis.
Dr W Osler 1904

The case history interview is a combination of the formal verbal investigation of the patient's symptoms and the observation of any subtle signs that may assist in the building of a complete picture of the patient sitting in your treatment room. Throughout the whole of this process, an ever-changing working hypothesis will be generated, challenged and reviewed either from the patient telling the history of their problem, their replies to specific questions from the practitioner or changes in their posture. Finally, when this working hypothesis cannot be further challenged by questioning, an initial diagnosis can be reached.

The taking of a careful and detailed case history will identify:-

- the likely tissue causing the patient's symptoms;
- the presence of any red flag conditions or contraindications to the physical examination or treatment;
- why the patient has developed this problem and to enable a practical treatment plan to be developed;
- the various psychosocial and environmental issues confronting the patient that will influence the treatment plan or the treatment outcome.

The process of taking a history begins immediately the patient has been identified to the practitioner. During this initial period, the practitioner will make several instinctive judgements, some relevant, unfortunately, most irrelevant or incorrect.

The observant practitioner may glean from this first interaction, before the formal case history process begins, enough information to formulate a very vague working hypothesis. This may be based upon the age of the patient, their static or active posture and their gait. **HOWEVER**, it is important to remember that the conditions that are obvious may **NOT** be what the patient wants addressed. The absence of such a hypothesis at this early stage should not be viewed as a failure, as a hastily ill-conceived hypothesis could prejudice the case history conclusions. It is prudent to use any information gleaned to rule out what the patient cannot, or is very unlikely to have, rather than what they do have.

Classically, a case history begins with the patient telling their story; they are the one suffering and by listening carefully to this history, the tissue or tissues causing the symptoms become apparent. The practitioner will use the natural breaks in the patient's dialogue to ask relevant open questions that will clarify specific aspects of the history. The more competent practitioner will have a flexible thought process that permits a working hypothesis to be generated, challenged, developed and modified as the history progresses from the current problem to past and current medical history. Eventually this hypothesis will identify one or more possible tissues causing symptoms and an initial diagnosis can be made. These tissues should be listed together with any specific tests or investigations the practitioner needs to undertake or arrange in order to reach a final diagnosis.

If this initial diagnosis identifies a possible visceral or medical cause of the patient's symptoms, a decision must be made whether to begin with the physical examination or refer the patient to their general practitioner. If the decision is made to continue, the practitioner must be willing to stop if it becomes self-evident that they are not competent to carry out the required examination or treat the tissues identified as causing the symptoms. When referral is necessary, the patient should be sent away satisfied with support, advice and, if necessary, a letter for their doctor.

The following flow chart, Figure 1.1, is an attempt to demonstrate the general thought processes that take place whilst taking a case history. It is an attempt to encourage the practitioner to think and ask specific questions that will enable the complete picture to develop rather than ask questions from a list or plucked from the air. Questions should be asked for a logical reason, in an order usually determined by the patient telling the history of their problem. The patient will respond and relax if the

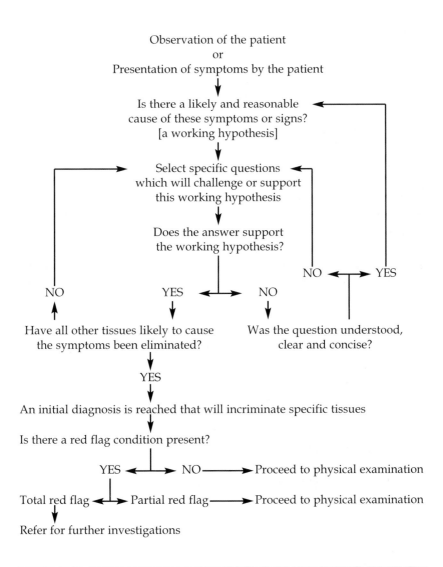

practitioner demonstrates an interest in them by asking questions using language the patient understands that relates to what has been said up to that time in the consultation.

Figure 1.1 Flow chart depicting some of the thought processes present during the taking of a case history.

Red flags and contraindications to treatment

A red flag condition can be defined as any condition that if left uninvestigated or untreated would be detrimental to the patient's general wellbeing. These conditions can be divided into two groups: the total red flag conditions that require immediate referral and treatment, and partial red flag conditions that require investigation in the near future. When deciding if a condition is a total or partial red flag, the prudent practitioner will always err on the side of caution.

Although the practitioner will always be alert for red flag conditions the commonest two contraindications to examination and treatment are the absence of consent from the patient or the absence of an initial diagnosis following the case history.

In brief, a red flag pathology should be suspected when the patient complains of:-

◆ severe unremitting pain or waves of pain;
◆ a deep constant ache or throbbing;
◆ severe night pain, sleep disturbed by pain;
◆ severe pain with no history of trauma or injury;
◆ pain unaffected by medication or position;
◆ a severe spasm or unusual protective posture;
◆ a bizarre symptom picture;
◆ symptoms related to specific systemic systems;
◆ unexplained fever, weight loss, generalised weakness or skin rashes, pallor or jaundice.

The facing page shows a table [Table 1] with a selection of symptoms that can be associated with a variety of systemic problems probably indicating the presence of either a total or partial red flag condition.

Table 1 A selection of symptoms associated with a variety of systemic problems.

Symptoms	Problem area
Persistent night pain, constant unremitting pain, unexplained weight loss, loss of appetite, unwarranted fatigue, rapid development or change of lumps, growths or moles	Cancer [any]
Muscle pain or weakness, specific red hot swollen joints, skin rash or adverse reaction to sunlight, nail or nail bed changes	Rheumatological
Headaches, vision changes, vertigo, seizures, loss of consciousness, poor coordination, weakness or atrophy of muscles, involuntary movements, tremor, paraesthesia, radicular pain, tinnitus, changes to hearing, swallowing, speech or balance	Neurological
Chest discomfort/pain, palpitations, pulsations anywhere in the body, peripheral oedema, claudication, deep pain in the calf, persistent cough, dyspnoea, syncope, shortness of breath, breathless at night lying flat, fatigue, nocturia	Cardiovascular
Heartburn, difficulty swallowing, nausea/vomiting, abdominal pain, indigestion, changes in bowel habit, diarrhoea, melaena, rectal bleeding, skin rash leading to joint pain	Gastrointestinal
Frequency, burning pain on passing water, reduced stream, reduced output, change in colour of urine, blood in urine, incontinence, impotence, nocturia, testicular pain	Genitourinary
Irregular monthly cycle, dysmenorrhoea, vaginal discharge, spotting between cycles, pain on intercourse, recent birth/termination, previous surgery, early menopause	Gynaecological
Hoarseness, cough, haemoptysis, shortness of breath, wheezing, night sweats, pleural pain, clubbing of fingers	Respiratory
Changes in hair or nails, intolerance of temperature changes, oedema, polydipsia, cramps, unexplained weakness, fatigue, generalised paraesthesia	Endocrine
Clusters of several different symptoms lasting more than one month, sleep disturbances, high stress levels, fatigue, psychomotor agitation, change in personal habits or appetite, depression, anxiety, confusion	Psychiatric
Skin or nail bed colour change, bleeding nose or gums, easily bruised, haemarthrosis, weakness, fatigue, dyspnoea, confusion, irritability, headaches	Haematological
Bone fracture, severe lacerations, severe shock, night sweats, fever [including flu], severe sore throat, recent severe emotional or physical upset, transient or constant swelling in one or more joints without injury, unexplained changes to general health or weight	Others

Figures 1.2 and 1.3 are an attempt to break down, by way of a flow chart, the challenging process of reaching an initial diagnosis during the formal case history process where the symptoms arise from the vertebral column. In both scenarios the patient can be, and often is, incorrect in their assumption of the causative event. The following two flow charts are **NOT** designed to offer a short cut to diagnosis or to cover every combination of tissue injury but to give structure and logic to the practitioner's thought processes.

Figure 1.2 covers the scenario when the patient cannot identify a cause or reason for the onset of the symptoms. Although postural stress, occupational posture and emotional upsets will be factors in these conditions and will influence how the symptoms develop, they have not been directly incriminated in this scenario by the patient or from the case history. There will occasionally be differences in the daily symptom pattern between a work and leisure day.

Figure 1.3 covers the alternative scenario when the patient thinks they can identify an event which started the problem. These include the obvious lifting or rotational traumas, accidents and injuries. The onset is often sudden, either in the recent or distant past, occurring at any time of the day. There is occasionally a daily pattern that can vary between a work day and rest or weekend day. It must be remembered that even with the simplest, most obvious conditions, there may be underlying long-term conditions present.

Even in this scenario where the patient identifies a precise causative event, the alert practitioner will be able to theorise about possible microtrauma or postural stress that underlie the problem which may prevent or delay the healing process.

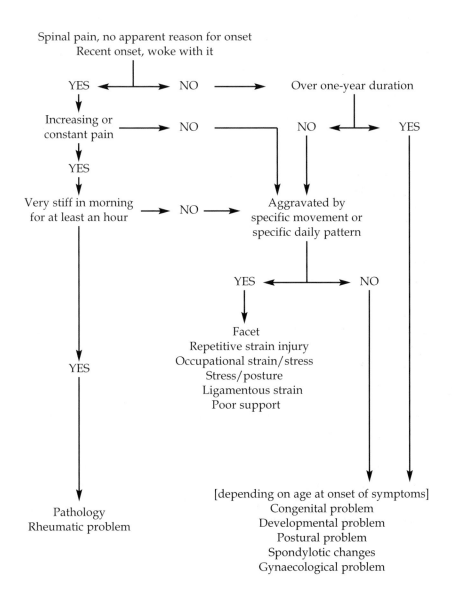

Figure 1.2 Flow chart depicting the challenging process of reaching an initial diagnosis during the formal case history process where the patient cannot identify a cause or reason for the onset of the symptoms.

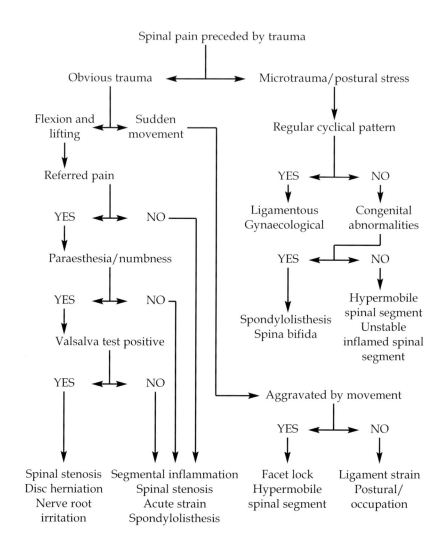

Figure 1.3 Flow chart depicting the challenging process of reaching an initial diagnosis during the formal case history process where the patient can identify a cause or reason for the onset of the symptoms.

Chapter 2

Physical examination

This formal physical examination of the patient should occur every time the patient presents for treatment, evaluation or re-assessment. Although it is the natural progression from the case history, it will only be performed when:-

♦   an initial diagnosis has been reached as to the tissue or tissues causing symptoms;
♦   a physical examination is indicated;
♦   there are no contraindications or total red flag conditions present.

As the physical examination of the patient begins, the initial working diagnosis is put aside and a new working hypothesis generated, challenged and amended. This enables the examination to begin afresh, without a pre-determined outcome. The only aspect of the initial diagnosis that is used during the physical examination is the part identifying specific areas that need to be examined or tested. This may be a specific system or a particular tissue that was identified as the possible site of a pathological process. When the physical examination has been completed, the working hypothesis, as in the case history, will have been amended several times and a working diagnosis reached.

Throughout the physical examination, contemporaneous notes must be made together with schematic drawings noting all areas of asymmetry and points of interest. These are vital if, in the future, comparisons are to be made or, medical or legal reports written. As all the findings within the physical examination are subjective in nature and may be seen by different practitioners, clarity of notes, drawings and procedures is essential.

Figure 2.1 is very similar to the diagram used to illustrate the case history process and as such shows the practitioner's thought processes during the physical examination. It is purely a theoretical model and will not be applicable in its entirety in the clinical setting.

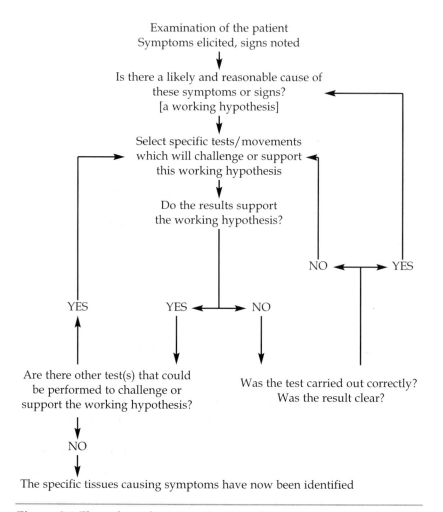

Figure 2.1 Flow chart depicting the thought processes present during the physical examination routine.

The physical examination process can be broken down into seven separate stages. The first four stages will be performed in a routine adapted by the individual practitioner on every patient. The following three stages - active resisted movements, the special orthopaedic and other special tests - will only be included if necessary.

1. Observation [standing, sitting and lying].
2. Palpation of the soft tissues and bony landmarks [standing, sitting and lying].
3. Active movements.
4. Passive articulation.
5. Active resisted movements.
6. Special orthopaedic or functional tests.
7. Other tests: neurological, cardiovascular, respiratory or specific system examination procedure.

The first four stages should follow a simple pattern progressing from the general to the specific and should be carried out in all planes of the body. The next three stages, if required, will be tissue-specific and conducted symmetrically initially on the symptom-free side using a routine that is designed to test all aspects of that selected system.

1. Observation

Throughout the consultation, from their arrival to departure, the ease with which the patient moves, sits, undresses and manoeuvres is noted. The practitioner compares these observations with the claimed aggravating and relieving features from the case history and notes any inconsistencies. There are many reasons why inconsistencies occur. They can simply be due to the patient's misunderstanding of a question, exaggerating the level of pain in an effort to be taken seriously, wanting to gain time off work or, more seriously, building a strong fraudulent case for an insurance claim. During the physical examination, the practitioner makes a subjective record of the patient's posture in the lateral and anterior-posterior planes noting any asymmetries together with the position of the centre of gravity, skin blemishes, scars, moles or areas of callus.

2. Palpation

Although not strictly palpation, the skin temperature should be assessed by placing the dorsum of the hand just above the skin. Palpation should always begin superficially with the practitioner noting the skin texture, degree of perspiration, and intensity of the red reaction. As palpation becomes deeper, the practitioner assesses and notes the tone and symmetry of the superficial and deeper muscles before palpating and noting the relative positions of the bony landmarks. The practitioner should reflect on whether the findings from palpation support the findings noted when observing the patient. If not, a hypothesis for the difference should be generated.

3. Active movements

These are performed within the pain-free range, in a routine designed to test paired movements. It is important to note the range of active pain-free movement and what, pain or tissue, limits the movement. Any accessory movements should be noted and all findings subjectively noted for future comparison.

4. Passive articulation

As the term suggests, the joints are taken through their full pain-free range of movement by the practitioner, starting with the pain-free side. Subjective comparisons are drawn between the two sides [additionally in the spine between adjacent segments] and compared with the expected normal physiological range for someone of the same age and sex.

Every joint that is controlled by muscles (**NOT** the sacroiliac or inferior tibiofibular joint) has a unique pattern of limitation or restriction.

Loose packed position
The position of maximum tissue laxity, with the minimum congruency between the articular surfaces. It is the usual position of rest for the joint.

Close packed position
The position of maximum tissue tension, with the maximum congruency between the articular surfaces. This reduces the normal accessory movements and places the joint in compression.

5. Active resisted movements

The joint is placed in the mid-range of movement and the patient instructed to resist the graded directional forces applied by the practitioner. As a general rule the pain-free limb is tested first. This, by alerting the patient to what is expected, will enhance patient relaxation, reduce fear of the unexpected and clarify the test results.

6. Orthopaedic or functional tests

These should only be conducted to confirm a hypothesis or for practice rather than used as a screening routine. They are performed bilaterally, on the pain-free side first, to allow direct comparison between 'normal' and 'abnormal' sides. All findings, including negative ones, should be noted. Great care needs to be exercised particularly when undertaking instability tests and the patient's wellbeing must be considered before undertaking the test.

7. Specific system examination

The examination of specific systems should not be used as a screening routine but to confirm a hypothesis, rule out a visceral cause of the patient's symptoms, or to practise the routine. The neurological examination is performed bilaterally, on the pain-free side first. The other systems should be examined with a routine that begins away from the area of the symptoms before moving towards the sensitive area. All findings, including negative ones, should be noted.

During the physical examination process it is important to remember that:-

♦ some tests needed to confirm a diagnosis may be beyond the ability of the practitioner either due to inexperience or lack of specialised equipment;
♦ some tests may be **DANGEROUS** to perform, especially the instability tests.

Once a working diagnosis has been generated from the physical examination, it should correspond and support the original working diagnosis reached after the case history. If there are marked discrepancies, the practitioner should review the findings from the case history and physical examination before the commencement of treatment.

If both working diagnoses correspond, the practitioner can formulate a final working diagnosis. This will identify the tissues causing symptoms, subjectively comment upon specific dysfunction within the joints and tissues and note any psychosocial and environmental factors that may have a bearing on the patient's short and long-term prognosis. Although an overall treatment plan is devised, it will be reviewed and modified at each subsequent treatment as the patient's symptoms, activities and circumstances change.

It is important to note that this final diagnosis although phrased in medical terminology is purely an educated guess based upon the information available at the time and as such is fluid and is subject to change when more information becomes available.

Chapter 3

Postural analysis

How a patient's posture develops and deviates from a perceived perfect example under the constant influences of life, the universe and everything is reviewed in this chapter. A good posture can be defined as one which is balanced, places the minimal stress on individual tissues and uses the minimum amount of energy to maintain. The detailed assessment of the patient's posture is essential if the practitioner is to understand how the patient defies the constant forces of gravity, and to understand some of the factors that have contributed to their current problem. In addition, information is gained that will influence the immediate and long-term treatment plan and give an indication to the likelihood of the problem recurring. In this respect it could be argued that the analysis of the patient's posture is the most important aspect of the consultation process.

Before the postural observation process is outlined, it is prudent to recognise some of the many factors - congenital, developmental, traumatic, habitual or pathological - that can influence how a posture develops. Some of the more obvious ones are listed below.

Congenital

This group includes any condition that develops before or becomes apparent just after birth and includes cerebral palsy, congenital dislocation of the hip, and hemivertebra.

Developmental

This large group includes the asymmetrical growth of various structures or specific failure of bony fusion [spondylolysis]; imbalances that are triggered by hormonal changes [adolescent pregnancy or post-menopausal]; the changing habits, physical activities, psychosocial pressures and body weight of the individual.

A few examples of how these factors at different ages can affect the patient are listed below. This is by no means a complete list.

The infant
Babies put into a cot in the same position every time will lift their head in response to sound, using and developing specific muscles that could become over-developed. This will lead to the neck muscles exerting an asymmetrical pull on the soft developing vertebrae.

The toddler
The toddler imitates the different postures or habits of their parents or carers.

The child
The carrying of heavy school bags on one shoulder can increase the strength of specific muscles placing an asymmetrical strain on the spine.

The teenager
The age that hormones are activated will, in girls, determine when breasts develop, which can affect the way a young girl stands. Teenagers are prone to sudden growth spurts, the bones rapidly lengthen and the muscle strength slowly develops putting the joints at risk of postural strain. The typical teenage slouch can precede a poor postural adaptation in adulthood.

The young adult
Prolonged periods of inactivity either at the computer or in the college lecture room. Poor nutrition due to low student income or lack of parental control will affect general health.

The adult
Many factors will affect this large age group including pregnancy, weak abdominal muscles and a pronounced beer belly.

The middle-aged adult
Optimistic expectations of their physical capabilities linked with the natural degeneration process of joints, ligaments and muscles.

The elderly adult
A more sedentary lifestyle, an unwillingness to change habits of a lifetime or use mobility aids.

Traumatic

Any traumatic episode or bony fracture will generate a specific compensatory mechanism to develop whilst healing occurs. How the body returns to normal function after the healing process has been completed will have a long-term impact on the development of symptoms locally and distally.

Habitual

Any habitual or asymmetrical posture, the wearing of fashionable shoes, or specific asymmetrical leisure pursuits, will develop the strength of unbalanced muscle groups so impacting on the overall balance of the body.

Pathological

There are many pathological processes that will affect how a posture develops, initially or in later life, and they will influence how the body functions or how its nutritional needs are met. Some of the commonest are listed below:-

Respiratory system	Asthma, emphysema, smoking.
Gastrointestinal system	Crohn's disease, ulcerative colitis, malabsorbtion syndrome.
Musculoskeletal system	Joint disease or degeneration, Scheuermann's disease, idiopathic scoliosis.

Observation of the posture

The following routine covers the observation aspect of the standard standing examination mentioned in the previous chapter. However, it can be adapted when examining the patient sitting or lying.

As the patient is requested to undress to their underwear, great care should be taken to retain their dignity and put them at their ease as their normal posture only becomes apparent once they are relaxed. It is recommended that to preserve the patient's modesty, the initial observations should be conducted from behind, with a clear explanatory narrative encouraging the patient to stand in a comfortable position that, pain permitting, resembles their normal relaxed posture.

The patient's posture is compared to the perfect erect posture as viewed from behind [Figure 3.1] and viewed from the side [Figure 3.2].

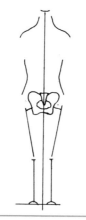

In the perfect erect posture when viewed from behind, the centre of gravity line begins in the midline at the atlas, passes through all vertebrae and the pelvis ending at a point mid way between the feet. The waist, buttock and knee creases would be level, as would the mastoid processes, shoulders, scapula and bony points of the pelvis. The centre of gravity of the body is just anterior to S2 in women, slightly higher in men, and lower in children.

Figure 3.1 The perfect erect posture when viewed from behind.

When viewed from the side in the perfect posture, a straight line dropped from the mastoid process would appear to pass through the shoulder joint, passing just posterior to the hip joint and just anterior to the knee, finally passing through the navicular bone. The bodies of the cervical and lumbar vertebrae should fall just on this imaginary line. The sacral base is at an angle of 30° to the horizontal.

When standing with a perfect posture, the natural movement of each area as indicated by the arrows is resisted by the structures named.

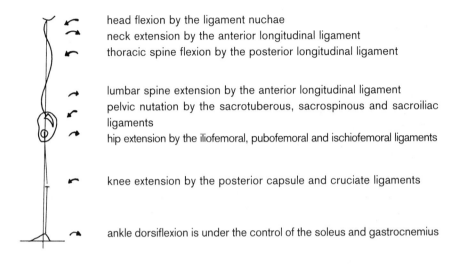

head flexion by the ligament nuchae

neck extension by the anterior longitudinal ligament

thoracic spine flexion by the posterior longitudinal ligament

lumbar spine extension by the anterior longitudinal ligament

pelvic nutation by the sacrotuberous, sacrospinous and sacroiliac ligaments

hip extension by the iliofemoral, pubofemoral and ischiofemoral ligaments

knee extension by the posterior capsule and cruciate ligaments

ankle dorsiflexion is under the control of the soleus and gastrocnemius

Figure 3.2 The perfect erect posture when viewed from the side.

In observing the patient, the first task is to decide if their current posture in either plane is protective, functional or habitual:-

- **A protective posture** is one adopted in response to a specific injury protecting that tissue to the detriment of others. These are extreme, unstable, likely to change during the observation process and are accompanied by overt muscle spasm and pain;
- **A functional posture** is temporary and reversible and is adopted to enable the body to complete a specific task or job with the minimum expenditure of energy. The normal posture will return once that task has been completed or after a period of rest;
- **A habitual posture** is the one the patient normally adopts while standing, sitting, walking or lying. As the habitual posture is constantly subjected to different stresses and strains relating to the patient's age, weight changes, occupation or lifestyle, it is modified, amended and altered throughout life.

Hands on: a clinical companion

When viewing from behind, any lateral deviation of the spine is defined as a scoliosis and can be described as an 'S' or a 'C' scoliosis, with the side of the convexity naming the scoliosis. In Figures 3.3 and 3.4 a 'C' and an 'S' scoliosis convex right in the lumbar spine are shown with the tissues that are tightened [parallel lines], weakened [wavy lines] and shortened [horizontal lines] identified.

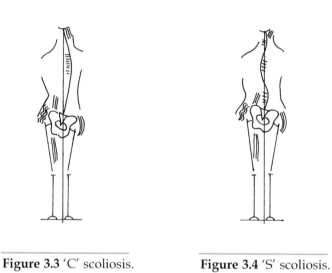

Figure 3.3 'C' scoliosis.　　　　**Figure 3.4** 'S' scoliosis.

When viewing from the side, any anterior-posterior increase in curvature of the spine from the perfect shape is named after the curve that has had the major change applied, accepting all curves will be affected to some degree. An increase in the thoracic curve will be termed a kyphosis [Figure 3.5], in the lumbar spine a lordosis [Figure 3.6] or sway back [Figure 3.7]. Where the spine has reduced curvature, the term used is a flat back [Figure 3.8]

These postures will only be maintained by asymmetrical changes in the muscles or ligamentous tissue. In the following diagrams, the tissues that are tightened [parallel lines], weakened [wavy lines] and shortened [horizontal lines] are identified as they place different stresses onto the underlying joints and support structures.

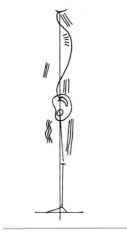

There is an increased angular change at the cervicodorsal junction, protracted shoulders with a shortened pectoralis major and serratus anterior.

The kyphosis extends into the upper lumbar spine and the sacral base makes a 20° angle with the horizontal.

Figure 3.5 Kyphosis.

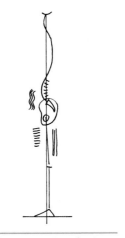

The lumbar facets take more weight leading to articular problems, particularly at the lumbosacral, sacroiliac, dorsolumbar and hip joints. The sacral base makes a 40° angle to the horizontal.

If there is a pes planus or the hips are held habitually in external rotation, this posture can develop.

Figure 3.6 Lordosis.

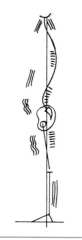

The head is carried forward of the centre of gravity placing strain on the cervical muscles. The kyphosis extends into the upper lumbar spine; the remaining lordosis is deep and short. The hips and knees are held in an excessive degree of extension.

The pelvis is thrust and rotated anteriorly with the sacral base angle of 40° to the horizontal.

Figure 3.7 Sway back.

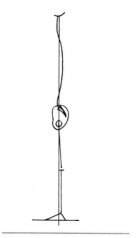

The kyphosis is long and shallow leading to a short sharp lordosis with reduced mobility.

The sacral base makes an angle of only 20° with the horizontal.

Figure 3.8 Flat back.

Leg length discrepancy

As leg length discrepancies will influence the patient's posture a subjective assessment of the relative leg lengths should be made on every patient, no matter the original complaint. This should be conducted initially with the patient standing relaxed, adopting their usual stance, standing 'at attention' and lying supine. In this context 'at attention' is when the patient stands with the feet together, knees fully extended, and toes facing straight ahead. It is important to ensure that this position is adopted, as a functional short leg can immediately be induced if the hip is placed in medial rotation, the knee flexed or the foot pronated.

When the patient is standing, the differences in leg length is determined by comparing the relative positions of the pelvic bony landmarks; superiorly, the iliac crest; anteriorly, the anterior superior iliac spine [ASIS]; and posteriorly, the posterior superior iliac spine [PSIS].

The following initial assumptions can then be made:-

♦ PSIS up, crest and ASIS down indicate an anteriorly rotated innominate on that side or a posteriorly rotated innominate on the other side;
♦ PSIS, crest and ASIS down indicate a short leg on that side, or long leg on the other side.

Functional differences in leg length between standing relaxed and 'at attention' are very common. When standing relaxed the pelvis is often level; this is achieved by adopting a different degree of hip abduction, flexion or rotation, knee flexion or foot supination or pronation. These subtle changes are removed when standing 'at attention' and allow an accurate assessment of the leg length discrepancy to be made.

When the patient is lying supine on the treatment table, an initial assessment of the leg lengths is made. The practitioner palpates the medial malleoli, noting differences in relative height and compares this with the relative position of the ASIS. The patient is then asked to flex both knees to 45°, lift their pelvis off the treatment table and carefully relax back onto the table. With the knees still flexed the practitioner can see any obvious leg length discrepancy by noting the relative positions of the patellae or tibial tuberosities. The knees are passively extended and with the patient lying flat, feet together, the relative positions of the medial malleoli and ASISs are again noted.

The following assumptions can be made from these relative positions:-

♦ If the malleoli are level and the ASIS is down [or the ASIS level and malleolus up], there is a short leg on that side, or long leg on the opposite side.
♦ If both points are up, ASIS and medial malleolus, it may indicate the patient is lying slightly twisted or the pelvis is being held rotated.

The findings from both the standing and lying examination are compared and if different, a hypothesis for the difference should be formulated.

Chapter 4

The cervical spine

Although the cervical spine comprises seven vertebrae, functionally they can be divided into two groups, the suboccipital comprising the atlas and axis, and the remaining five.

A typical cervical vertebra [Figure 4.1] consists of a body with a unciform process projecting superiorly from the lateral borders and a slight anterior and posterior ledge.

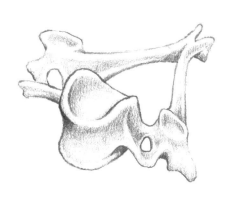

The pedicles are attached to the posterior aspect of the lateral border of the body and give rise anteriorly to the transverse process and posteriorly to the articular process. The transverse process is perforated by the foramen transversarium for the vertebral artery and ends with two tubercles for the attachment of the scalene muscles. The articular process bears the articular facets and gives rise, posteriorly, to the laminae which meet posteriorly in the midline to form the bifid spinous process.

Figure 4.1 A typical cervical vertebra.

In the suboccipital area, the first cervical vertebra, the atlas [Figure 4.2], is a ring of bone with two pairs of articular surfaces forming two lateral masses. Upon the anterior arch is a small articular facet for articulation with the odontoid peg of the axis and in the midline of the posterior arch is a posterior tubercle.

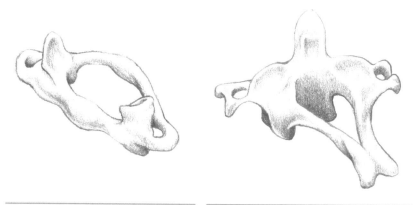

Figure 4.2 The atlas.   **Figure 4.3** The axis.

The second cervical vertebra, the axis [Figure 4.3], is similar to the typical cervical vertebrae except for the odontoid peg that projects from the superior surface of the body and articulates with the posterior surface of the anterior arch of the atlas.

Ligaments of the cervical spine

Suboccipital complex

The shape of the paired synovial joints between the atlas and occipital condyles allows practically no rotation or side-bending, only limited flexion and extension - a slight nodding of the head. In addition to the capsule of the atlanto-occipital joints, there is the thin fibrous atlanto-occipital membrane attaching the occiput to the atlas. This membrane is pierced by the vertebral artery as it progresses superiorly and by the 1st cervical nerve.

Between the atlas and axis there are three synovial joints, the paired atlanto-axial joints and the articulation between the odontoid peg and the posterior surface of the anterior arch of the atlas. This articulation allows over 50% of cervical rotation to occur whilst preventing any other movements.

The odontoid peg is held securely in place by the cruciform ligament. The stronger transverse bands run between the two lateral masses of the atlas. Slightly superficial to this is the tectorial membrane, the superior extension of the posterior longitudinal ligament that had its origin at the level of the sacrum. Attached to the odontoid peg are the paired alar ligaments that fan superiorly and laterally to the occiput. In addition, there is an apical ligament that attaches to the occiput in the midline. These ligaments restrict rotation and ensure that the odontoid peg and atlas remain in close approximation.

The other ligaments of the cervical spine comprise:-

Anterior longitudinal ligament
This is a broad band on the anterior and anterior-lateral surfaces of the vertebral bodies, extending from the atlas to the sacrum. The fibres are firmly attached to the anterior margins of the vertebral bodies.

Posterior longitudinal ligament
This runs within the vertebral canal. In the cervical spine it is broad. It is firmly attached to the vertebral margins, but separated by loose connective tissue from the bodies, allowing blood vessels easy access to the vertebrae.

Ligamentum flava
These are the strongest and most important paired posterior ligaments within the cervical spine. They run between the lamina of adjacent vertebrae.

Ligamentum nuchae
This is a strong thick elastic band that assists in holding the head upright. Stretching from the external occipital protuberance to the spinous process of the 7th cervical vertebra, it offers a point of attachment to the trapezius.

Interspinous ligaments
These are deep to the ligamentum nuchae and run between adjacent spinous processes.

Intertransverse ligaments
These run between adjacent transverse processes.

Intervertebral disc

These are between all the vertebral bodies, except the atlas and axis. Each disc comprises a central gelatinous part, the nucleus pulposus situated slightly within the posterior portion of the disc and a fibrous covering, the annulus fibrosus. The fibres of the annulus are arranged in concentric circles, like the layers of an onion. However, each layer has a different slant to the preceding one, increasing the strength of the structure without limiting its flexibility. Signs of degeneration are apparent from the third decade and result in microcracks forming between the layers weakening the whole structure.

Muscles of the cervical spine

The muscles of the neck can be divided into superficial and deep. They are paired and depending upon their individual contractions, can induce different movements. They can be broadly split into two functional groups, those that have an effect upon the position of the head and those that have an effect upon the position of the neck [Table 1].

Table 1 The muscles of the cervical spine.

Position of the head, maintained by the deep muscles

Flexion	Rectus capitis anterior, longus colli, mylohyoid, longus capitis
Extension	Obliquis capitis superior, rectus capitis posterior minor and major
Side-bending	Rectus capitis lateralis
Ipsilateral rotation	Obliquis capitis superior, rectus capitis post major, obliqus capitis inferior

Position of the neck

	Superficial muscles	Deep muscles
Flexion	Scalenus posterior, sternocleidomastoid	Longus colli, longus capitis
Extension	Levator scapulae	Spinalis, longissimus, semispinalis, splenius, iliocostalis
Side-bending	Scalenus anterior and posterior, levator scapulae, sternocleidomastoid	Spinalis, longissimus, semispinalis, splenius, iliocostalis
Rotation	**Contralateral** Scalenus posterior, sternocleidomastoid	**Ipsilateral** Spinalis, longissimus, semispinalis, splenius

For a diagrammatic representation of the muscles, see Figures 4.4 and 4.5. Tables 2 and 3 list the muscles, and give a brief description of their origin and insertion. The erector spinae muscles and deep segmental muscles are described in the muscle section of Chapter 6 - The lumbar spine.

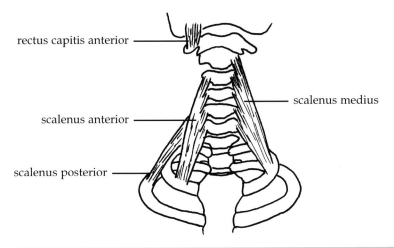

Figure 4.4 The anterior muscles of the cervical spine.

Table 2 The anterior muscles of the cervical spine.

	Origin	Insertion
Longus capitis/colli	T/P anterior body C3-6	Same several segments up
Rectus capitis anterior	T/P atlas	Anterior foramen magnum
Scalenus		
anterior	T/P anterior tubercle C3-6	1st rib
medius	T/P posterior tubercle C2-7	1st rib
posterior	T/P posterior tubercle C4-6	2nd and 3rd rib
Sternocleidomastoid	Sternum and clavicle	Mastoid process

Footnote
S/P = Spinous Process   T/P = Transverse Process
The abbreviations above are used in tables throughout the entire book.

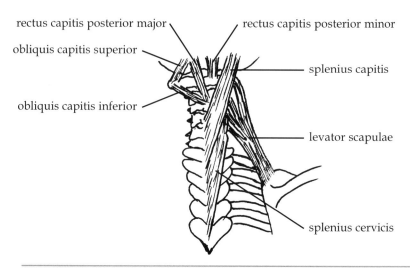

rectus capitis posterior major

rectus capitis posterior minor

obliquis capitis superior

splenius capitis

obliquis capitis inferior

levator scapulae

splenius cervicis

Figure 4.5 The posterior muscles of the cervical spine.

Table 3 The posterior muscles of the cervical spine.

	Origin	Insertion
Obliquis capitis inferior	S/P axis	T/P atlas
Obliquis capitis superior	T/P atlas	Between nuchal lines
Rectus capitis posterior major	S/P axis	Inferior nuchal line
Rectus capitis posterior minor	Posterior tubercle of atlas	Inferior nuchal line
Splenius capitis	S/P C3-T4	Superior nuchal line
Splenius cervicis	S/P T3-6	T/P C2-4
Iliocostalis cervicis	Angles ribs 1-6	T/P C4-6
Longissimus capitis	Articular pillars C4-7	Mastoid process
Longissimus cervicis	T/P T1-6	T/P C2-6
Spinalis capitis	S/P low Cs, upper Ts	Between nuchal lines
Spinalis cervicis	S/P C6-T2	S/P C2
Semispinalis capitis	T/P T1-6; articular pillars, C4-7	Between nuchal lines
Semispinalis cervicis	T/P T1-6	S/P C2-T5
Levator scapulae	T/P C1-4	Superior angle scapula

Differential diagnosis in the cervical spine

Tables 4 and 5 are not designed to be the means to a definite diagnosis for the commonest cervical musculoskeletal problems but rather to identify the commonest and classical symptoms associated with each condition. It is important to remember that every patient is unique; how they react to and interpret their symptoms provides the practitioner with the challenge of making a diagnosis. For ease, the various causes have been divided into impingement conditions and degenerative conditions.

Table 4 Common impingement conditions.

Signs/symptoms	Facet	Nerve root	Thoracic outlet
Age at onset [yrs]	Any	Any	Any
Mode of onset	Sudden	Sudden	Insidious
Pain site	Localised, unilateral	Localised, unilateral	Generalised over trapezius
Pain/paraesthesia referral	Possible	To one dermatome	Via affected nerves
Aggravating features	Ipsilateral movement, extension	Ipsilateral side-bending or extension	Prolonged neck flexion, carrying
Relieving features	Heat, immobility	Contralateral side-bending	Gentle mobility support
Special tests	Spurling's	Spurling's, brachial plexus tension test	Adson's

Other nerves that can be irritated in the cervical spine are the vagus and the sympathetic chain from the thoracic spine.

There are three ganglions from the sympathetic chain within the cervical spine:-

- stellate ganglion between C7 and 1st rib, lateral to longus colli;
- middle cervical ganglion [may be absent], at C6 on longus colli;
- superior cervical ganglion, the largest at C2-3, on longus capitis.

Generally, over-stimulation can lead to inhibited healing, affect immune and allergic reactions and adversely affect the rate and rhythm of the heart.

Table 5 Common degenerative conditions.

Signs/symptoms	Spondylosis	Stenosis	Disc herniation
Age at onset [yrs]	Most over 60	Commonest 30-70	Commonest 17-40
Mode of onset	Insidious	Insidious	Sudden traumatic
Pain site	Generalised	Variable	Localised spasm
Pain/paraesthesia referral	Possible dermatomal	Several dermatomes	Dermatomal
Aggravating features	Static upright posture, movement to limit	Extension of neck movement	Heavy lifting, pressure, flexion
Relieving features	Gentle mobility, heat	Gentle flexion of neck	Rest, support
Special tests	X-ray	X-ray	Spurling's

Degenerative changes in the cervical spine can, by virtue of the development of a cervical bar, cause cervical stenosis. When a stenosis is present, the reflexes with origins above the level are normal, but with an origin below can be increased, depending on the damage or constriction of the spinal cord.

Common pathological conditions of the cervical spine

Deformities

Spondylolysis
This can occur at C1/2 due to a congenital absence of the ligaments around the odontoid peg, a failure of fusion of the odontoid peg, instability of the odontoid peg in rheumatoid arthritis, or following injury. If suspected **EXTREME** care should be exercised when examining the neck; it should **NEVER** be placed into extension.

Cervical rib

A congenital abnormality; either an osseous or a thickened fibrous band. The symptoms arise from an irritation of vessels or nerves passing over the rib with symptoms radiating into the upper limb. They may be due to irritation of the sympathetic outflow [increased sweating in the hand], or an impingement of the vascular supply [reduced pulses]. The neurological symptoms may not be limited to a single nerve or nerve root.

Torticollis

This is caused by contracture of the sternocleidomastoid. Often seen in children up to 3 years of age but also in adults. Before a positive diagnosis can be made, the other causes - infected glands, deformity of the cervical spine, or hysterical torticollis - must be ruled out. The presence of facial deformity or asymmetry will give an indication of the condition's duration.

Klippel-Feil syndrome

A congenital short neck with bony deformities and general mobility restriction of the neck with segmental fusions present.

Sprengel's shoulder

A congenital high scapula which can be unilateral or bilateral, resulting in a general restriction of all ranges of movement of the scapula.

Infections

Pyogenic

This is uncommon and is spread via blood or lymph. There will be signs of pyrexia and symptoms from the original site of infection.

Tuberculosis

Rare, but seen in children or the young adult. It spreads from other foci. The patient will present with a rigid neck and a possible abscess.

Arthritis

Rheumatoid arthritis

The neck is occasionally affected, especially C1-2 where it causes laxity around the odontoid peg. The neck is stiff, swollen and has a slight reduction in range of movement. There will be signs of the disease elsewhere.

Osteoarthritis
Particularly affects the low cervical spine, especially C5/6/7, with formation of osteophytes, a cervical bar and foraminal narrowing. Affects older patients frequently with other joints affected. X-rays will confirm presence.

Ankylosing spondylitis
Gradual onset from lower in the spine, affecting the cervical spine in 50% of cases. There are associated symptoms of stiffness, pain in the low back and pelvis, and a reduced thoracic cage expansion.

Mechanical

Disc prolapse or herniation
This is not as common as in the lumbar spine. Commonest at C5/6 and C6/7 and there is generally a history of injury with pain/stiffness and nerve root irritation.

Tumours

All may lead to cord compression, bone collapse and/or nerve involvement. Primary tumours, benign or malignant, are rare; secondaries are more common.

Bone
Malignant primary sarcoma, multiple myeloma. Malignant secondary carcinoma, sarcoma.

Cord
Meningioma, intradural neurofibroma.

Nerve
Neurofibroma.

Common extrinsic causes of symptoms

Head

Intracranial space-occupying lesions, migraine headaches. Eyes, ear, sinus, dental or temporomandibular problems.

Respiratory system

Pancoast tumour within the upper lobe of the lung, trachiobronchial irritation.

Vascular system

Vertebral artery impingement, subclavicular artery impingement, angina pectoris, aortic aneurysm.

Physical examination of the cervical spine

The primary bony landmark is the spinous process of C7, the most prominent within the neck.

Positions and patterns

Resting   slight extension
Close packed   full extension

Active range of movement

flexion   60°-80°   **rotation**   80°
extension 40°-70°   **side-bending** 45°

Special tests for the cervical spine

These are all provocative tests. Each test comprises several stages, with each more provocative and, once the symptoms have been reproduced, the test is deemed positive and concluded.

Vascular signs

Hautant's vertebral artery test

This is designed to differentiate between vertebral artery and auricular dizziness. The patient sits supported by the practitioner, with their shoulders flexed to 90°, hands supinated and eyes closed. If the arm position changes when the eyes close, it suggests that the dizziness is non-vascular. The patient is then asked to extend and rotate the neck to one then the other side, holding the position for 20 seconds. If dizziness occurs or arm position alters, it is an indication that symptoms are vascular.

Vertebral artery test

The patient is lying supine with their eyes open and head supported in the neutral position beyond the end of the table. The practitioner passively fully extends and side-bends the neck, adding rotation to the same side. This position is held for up to 20 seconds. A positive test will provoke the referring symptoms or cause nystagmus to occur.

Adson's thoracic outlet test

While the patient sits well supported on the table, the practitioner locates the radial pulse at the wrist. The patient rotates their head to the same side and extends the neck whilst the practitioner laterally rotates and extends the shoulder. The patient is asked to take and hold a deep breath. The disappearance of the pulse indicates a positive test.

Compression tests

(N.B. for patient comfort these tests can also be performed supine.)

Spurling's foraminal compression

The patient sits supported by the practitioner, who places the patient's neck in the neutral position and exerts a compressive force down through the head compressing the cervical spine. If no symptoms are produced the test is repeated first with extension then rotation to the side of pain. For the test to be positive, nerve irritation within the vertebral foramen or facet compression will cause radicular pain from the neck.

Reverse Spurling

This is conducted as above except that the neck is rotated away from painful side. This test is for muscle spasm and is positive when pain is caused in this position.

Distraction

While the patient is sitting and supported, the practitioner takes the weight of the head and applies gentle traction. The test is positive if the symptoms are reduced, indicating pressure upon the nerve root has been relieved.

Specific neural tests

Brachial plexus tension test

This test can be slightly modified to tension different nerves within the brachial plexus and should be performed on the symptom-free side first with the patient lying supine. The elements are always added in the following order:-

- ◆ shoulder positioned and held depressed to the table by the practitioner's hand;
- ◆ the required degree of shoulder abduction is added;
- ◆ the forearm, then wrist, then fingers and finally, the elbow are positioned.

As each element is introduced, more tension is applied to the neural tissue. Once the symptoms have been reproduced, the test is deemed positive and concluded. If all elements have been added and the test has produced minimal or no symptoms, further tension can be applied by contralateral side-bending of the cervical spine.

To specifically stress the median, ulnar and radial nerves, the joints of the upper limb should be placed in positions as indicated in Table 6.

Table 6 The placed positions of the joints of the upper limb to specifically stress the median, ulnar and radial nerves.

	Shoulder	Forearm	Wrist	Fingers	Ebow
Median nerve C5/6/7	Abducted 110°	Supinated	Extended	Extended	Extended
Ulnar nerve C8/T1	Abducted 10-90°	Supinated	Extended radial deviation	Extended	Flexed
Radial nerve C6/7/8	Abducted 10°	Pronated	Flexed ulnar deviation	Flexed	Extended

Chapter 5

The thoracic spine and ribs

The twelve vertebrae of the thoracic spine increase in size caudally to form the posterior border of the thoracic cavity. They provide attachments to the ribs and these together with the costal cartilages and sternum provide protection for the major organs of the body.

The typical thoracic vertebra [Figure 5.1], has a body that is proportionally higher than the lumbar vertebrae and roughly equal in the transverse and anterior-posterior dimensions, whilst the anterior-lateral surfaces are slightly concave or hollow. On the posterior-lateral aspect of the body are the paired superior and inferior oval costal articular facets [demifacets]; the superior facet often extends onto the root of the pedicle.

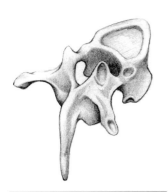

Figure 5.1 A typical thoracic vertebra.

The pedicle is strong and thick and arises from the upper part of the posterior surface of the body, resulting in a deep inferior vertebral notch. The vertebral foramen is smaller than the cervical and lumbar, and circular.

The laminae are broad and flat, overlapping the one below like tiles on a roof uniting in the midline to form the spinous process. On the superior border is the superior articular process and the flat oval articular facet. On the inferior border is the inferior articular process and corresponding facet.

Extending from the articular process is the transverse process, which faces slightly posteriorly and laterally. This is a strong thick structure with a thickened end with small concave articular facets for the rib. The spinous process is sharply inclined inferiorly; those of T5-8 extend to cover the next vertebrae, while that of T8 covers part of T10.

The first thoracic vertebra [Figure 5.2] and T9,10,11,12 [Figure 5.3] are modified slightly from the typical thoracic vertebra with the differences listed below.

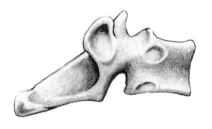

T1 is like the cervical vertebrae, being the same size as C7. The superior surface of the body is lipped laterally and the anterior border is bevelled. The inferior surface is flat like a typical thoracic vertebra.

Figure 5.2 T1.

The upper costal facet on the body is circular, the lower facet a demifacet. There are two vertebral notches and the spinous process is almost as prominent as C7.

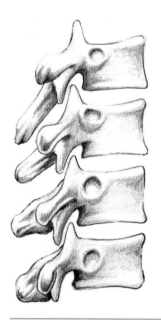

T9 often fails to articulate with the 10th rib so there is no inferior demifacet.

T10 has only a superior costal facet for the 10th rib. The transverse process may not have a facet for the rib.

T11 has only one costal facet for the 11th rib. The transverse process is small with no articular facet.

T12 is similar to a lumbar vertebra with regard to body size, pedicles, transverse and spinous processes. The 12th rib articulates with the middle of the body; the transverse process has superior, inferior and lateral tubercles. The superior articular facets are thoracic in shape whilst the inferior are lumbar in shape.

Figure 5.3 T9, T10, T11, T12.

There are twelve pairs of ribs, divided into three groups: true, false and floating.

True	Ribs 1-7 connect directly to the sternum by a costal cartilage.
False	Ribs 8-10 connect to the sternum via the costal margin.
Floating	Ribs 11-12. The anterior end is encased in the abdominal muscles.

Between the ribs are the intercostal spaces, deeper anteriorly than posteriorly. The ribs increase in length to the 7th rib while the downward slant increases to the 9th rib, when they become more horizontal.

A typical rib, the 3rd to the 9th, has a thin and flattened shaft and is slightly twisted along its long length with two ridges along the inferior surface, where the intercostal muscles attach. In a groove between these muscular attachments, the intercostal vessels and nerves run. At the posterior or vertebral end, the head of the rib has two facets divided by a transverse crest. These facets articulate with the demifacets on the thoracic vertebrae. The neck of the rib is anterior to the corresponding transverse process and at the junction between the neck and the shaft is a tubercle that has a small facet that articulates with the small facet on the corresponding transverse process. At the anterior end is a small depression in the tip for the articulation with the costal cartilage.

The costal cartilage is an elastic material that attaches the anterior end of the true ribs to the sternum, and the false ribs via the rib margin to the tip of the sternum. Along the length of the cartilage, a degree of torsion can occur and with the presence of costal cartilage, the movement of the ribs during respiration is enhanced.

The lateral end of the cartilage is shaped like a flattened cone that fits snugly into the small depression in the anterior end of the rib. A limited degree of lateral and vertical movement but no rotation is possible.

The medial end of the cartilage of the first seven ribs interlocks into a 'V'-shaped depression on the lateral side of the sternum. Although this 'V'-shaped depression is completely filled by cartilage, a small degree of movement can occur vertically. The other costal cartilages join the costal cartilage above to form the costal margin.

The cartilages are more flexible in youth and tend to ossify with age, leading to a loss of thoracic flexibility and respiratory efficiency.

Differences from the typical rib

1st rib	The shortest, and most curved. It is broad, flat and slopes down and forward. The head has a small almost circular facet to articulate with the body of T1. Superiorly there are large roughened areas for the attachment of the scalenus muscles.
2nd rib	Twice the length of the first. There is no twist in the shaft.
10th rib	The head has only one facet that articulates with T10 and the disc between T9 and T10.
11th, 12th rib	There is no neck or tubercle present, and only one large articular facet. The anterior ends are tipped with cartilage but end within muscle.

Ligaments of the thoracic spine and ribs

Ligaments of the thoracic spine can be divided into two groups concerning the vertebral joints and the costovertebral joints.

Posterior vertebral ligaments

Supraspinous ligament
This runs over the tips of the spinous processes and blends with the thin interspinous ligaments.

Interspinous ligament
Ill-defined but runs between the spinous process of one vertebra to the spinous process above.

Ligamentum flavum

This is a paired flat ligament that runs between adjacent laminae and blends with the joint capsule.

Posterior longitudinal ligament

Narrow over the body, this expands over the ends of the bodies and intervening disc. It is firmly attached to the ends of the bodies, but is separated from them by connective tissue that contains the blood vessels to and from the bone.

Anterior vertebral ligaments

Anterior longitudinal ligament

Firmly attached to the margins of the vertebra and disc and at its strongest in the midline.

Costovertebral ligaments [Figure 5.4]

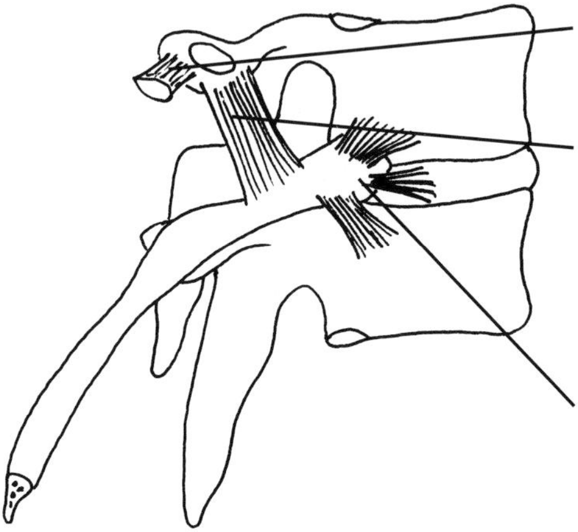

costotransverse ligament
[posterior, superior and inter-osseous bands]

posterior:
tip of transverse process to costal tubercle

superior:
transverse process to the underlying rib

interosseous:
transverse process to posterior neck of same rib, [not shown]

radiate ligament [three bands]
superior and inferior to adjacent vertebral bodies intermediate to annulus fibrosus of disc

interosseous ligament divides the rib articulation into two demifacets [not shown]

Figure 5.4 The costovertebral ligaments.

Intervertebral disc

These are between all the vertebral bodies except the atlas and axis. Each disc comprises a central gelatinous part, the nucleus pulposus situated slightly within the posterior portion of the disc, and a fibrous covering, the annulus fibrosus. The fibres of the annulus are arranged in concentric circles, like the layers of an onion. However, each layer has a different slant to the preceding one, increasing the strength of the structure without limiting its flexibility. Signs of degeneration are apparent from the third decade and result in microcracks forming between the layers weakening the whole structure.

Muscles of the thoracic spine and rib cage

The muscles of the thoracic spine are primarily concerned with respiration and posture; the mobility of the shoulder is a secondary concern. For details on the muscles controlling the shoulder, see Chapter 8 - The shoulder complex.

The thoracic muscles can be divided into deep and superficial. A more detailed description of the deep muscles can be found in Chapter 6 - The lumbar spine.

Diaphragm

This is a large muscle with a large central tendon and muscular fibres attaching to the costal cartilages, tips of ribs 11 and 12, the vertebral bodies via the crura, and medial surfaces of psoas and quadratus lumborum.

Contraction of the muscle initially uses the peripheral insertions, causing the central tendon to descend on to the abdominal contents. The central tendon then becomes stabilised by the abdominal contents and the continued muscular contraction acts to elevate the lower ribs.

Table 1 The muscles of the thoracic spine and ribs involved in inspiration and expiration. *Continued overleaf:-*

Superficial muscles of inspiration shown in Figure 5.5		
	Origin	**Insertion**
Sternocleidomastoid	Sternum and clavicle	Mastoid process
Scalenus		
anterior	T/P anterior tubercle C3-6	1st rib
medius	T/P posterior tubercle C2-7	1st rib
posterior	T/P posterior tubercle C4-6	2nd rib
Pectoralis major	Clavicle/sternum, upper 6 ribs	Lateral lip of bicipital groove
Pectoral minor	Ribs 2-5	Coronoid process
Serratus anterior	Upper 8/9 ribs	Medial margin scapula
Latissimus dorsi	S/P T7-L5, sacrum, iliac crest	Floor of bicipital groove
Serratus posterior superior	S/P C7-T2	Ribs 2-5

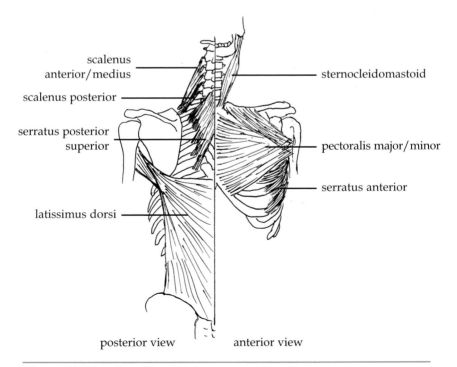

Figure 5.5 Muscles of inspiration.

Table 1 The muscles of the thoracic spine and ribs involved in inspiration and expiration. *Continued:-*

Deep muscles involved in inspiration

	Origin	Insertion
Iliocostalis superior fibres	Ribs 6-12	Rib angles 1-6, T/P C6-7
Levator costalis	T/Ps in thorax	Superior edge of rib below

Superficial muscles of expiration shown in Figure 5.6

Rectus abdominis	Pubis	Costal cartilage ribs 5-7 xiphoid process
External oblique	Lower 8 ribs	Iliac crest/pubis
Internal oblique	Rectus sheath, costal margin	Lumbar fascia, iliac crest
Quadratus lumborum	12th rib, T/P L1-4	Iliac crest
Serratus posterior inferior	S/P T11-L2	Posterior ribs 9-12

Deep muscles involved in expiration

Iliocostalis lower fibres	Upper border ribs 6-12	Lower border ribs 1-6
Longissimus thoracis	Sacrum, S/P T8-L5	Ribs near angle, lumbar spine T/Ps
Sternocostalis	Lower ½ inner sternum	Costal cartilages 2-6

Table 2 The other deep muscles of the thoracic spine and ribs.

	Origin	Insertion
Spinalis thoracis	S/P T10-12, L1-2	S/P T3- 9
Semispinalis thoracis	T/P T6-12	S/Ps of upper thoracic and low cervical
Multifidus	All T/Ps	S/Ps all vertebrae
Long/short rotators	All T/Ps	S/Ps all above
External intercostal	Inferior surface ribs	Superior surface of rib below
Internal intercostal	Superior surface ribs	Inferior surface of rib above

The exact function of the intercostal muscles in respiration is currently unclear.

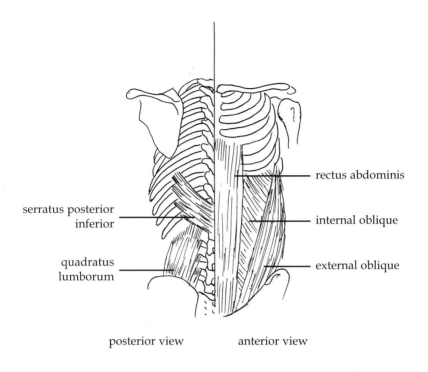

serratus posterior inferior

quadratus lumborum

rectus abdominis

internal oblique

external oblique

posterior view   anterior view

Figure 5.6 Muscles of expiration.

Common pathological conditions of the thoracic spine and ribs

Deformities

Scoliosis

Defined as any lateral plane curvature of the spine, no matter the cause. In idiopathic scoliosis occurring in 10-12 year old children, the treatment depends on severity and can require surgery or prolonged immobilisation. Other forms of scoliosis are either functional or protective and temporary in nature, or structural and permanent. Examples of causes of structural scoliosis are bony abnormality [hemivertebra], short leg, asymmetrical muscular development following polio or poor adaptive postures.

Kyphosis

An exaggerated normal anterior-posterior curvature of the thoracic spine is either congenital, developmental [poor posture], the result of an underlying disease process [tuberculosis, ankylosing spondylitis, tumour, osteochondrosis] or due to a fracture [trauma or osteoporosis].

Chest deformities

Pigeon chest A congenital condition where the sternum projects forward and down like the heel of a boot. Restricts ventilation volume.

Funnel chest A congenital condition where the sternum is pushed posteriorly by overgrowth of the ribs. The heart may be displaced, and the deformity may result in an increase in kyphosis. It will affect respiration.

Barrel chest The sternum projects up and anteriorly and develops in respiratory problems such as asthma and emphysema.

Osteoporosis

Common within the thoracic spine in petite, underweight, post-menopausal women, particularly when menopause is early. It can occur if there is a prolonged period of confinement to bed, in association with parathyroid osteodystrophy or Cushing's syndrome. Percussion is occasionally tender on the spinous processes and spontaneous unexplained fractures can occur leading to sudden marked reduction in height.

Scheuermann's vertebral osteochondritis

Develops in childhood between 13-16 years of age, possibly due to a disturbance within the normal development of the cartilage end plates and ring epiphyses of several vertebrae allowing disc material to herniate into the vertebral body. Generally within the thoracic spine and occasionally found in the upper lumbar spine. The active phase lasts about 2 years, and will result in a localised restriction of mobility of the affected vertebrae and occasionally localised pain.

Calvé's vertebral osteochondritis

This affects the central nucleus of one thoracic vertebral body. It is less common than Scheuermann's and mainly affects 2-10 year olds who complain of thoracic pain. There may be a slight increase in kyphosis and pain on percussion.

Infections

Pyogenic
This is uncommon and spreads via blood or lymph. There will be signs of pyrexia and symptoms from the original site of infection.

Tuberculosis
Attacks the anterior part of the vertebral body and disc, especially in young adults. It is, with the lumbar spine, the commonest site for tuberculosis. The patient looks ill and once the pain develops, firm palpation or percussion is tender locally with an overlying protective muscle spasm.

Arthritis

Rheumatoid arthritis
Occasionally affects the thoracic spine with stiffness, swelling and reduced mobility. However, there will be symptoms from other joints affected.

Osteoarthritis
Very common, particularly in the mature patient, although often symptom-free.

Ankylosing spondylitis
Gradually develops from below with an increase in kyphosis and reduced rib cage expansion. There will be gross restrictions in movement of the lumbar and thoracic spines.

Polymyalgia rheumatica
Especially in the 60+ age group, occurring in women three times as often as men. Occasionally, the patient can have similar symptoms in the pelvic girdle. The patient presents with morning stiffness that lasts for at least one hour. In the day the symptoms can return to normal with little stiffness or pain. A raised ESR is indicative, and corticosteroid therapy will clear the symptoms almost immediately. The condition will last for between 2-4 years requiring progressively less medication to control the symptoms.

Paget's disease
Dull aching pain aggravated by use or immobility, affecting men twice more often than women in the 40+ age group. Of unknown aetiology, it affects, in particular the pelvis, femur, skull, tibia and vertebrae.

Mechanical

Fractured rib
History of direct trauma to the area resulting in pain on breathing.

Costochondral joint strain
Following direct trauma or a severe cough/sneeze particularly in the mature patient. There is localised pain directly over the affected costochondral joint on taking a deep breath, or turning. It will slowly ease in 5-6 weeks.

Tumours

Bone
Metastatic carcinoma from the lung, breast, prostate, thyroid or kidney. Occasionally, primary tumours such as a sarcoma, multiple myeloma, or chondroma. The main local symptom is bone collapse.

Sternum
Blood-borne metastic tumours or deposits in myelomatosis.

Scapula
Chondroma; this grows outward and is classed as an ecchondroma when benign. However, it may become malignant.

Cord/nerve
Neurofibroma: symptoms depend upon site. There is girdle pain followed by lower motor signs, and bladder and bowel dysfunction.

Others

Herpes zoster
Unilateral pain followed by a rash 3-4 days later. It is confined to a single thoracic spinal dermatome.

Sympathetic chain irritation/stimulation
A chain of ganglia originating from the upper lumbar and thoracic spine providing 8% of spinal nerve tissue.

Generally fibres from:-

T1   go up to the head and neck via cervical ganglia.
T2   the neck and upper limb.
T3-6   the thorax.
T7-11   the abdomen.
T12   or below to the pelvis and lower limb.

Common extrinsic causes of symptoms

Heart

To the left or right shoulder and occasionally to the arm, neck or jaw.

Diaphragm

To the shoulder and C4 dermatome.

Abdominal disorders

Spleen to the left shoulder area; liver and gall bladder to the right shoulder area.

Lung and pleura

Pancoast tumour to the thoracic outlet area.

Renal disorders

To the 12th rib area.

Physical examination of the thoracic spine and ribs

Thoracic spine landmarks

Spinous process of T2   opposite the superior angle of the scapulae.
Spinous process of T3   opposite the root of the spine of the scapulae.
Spinous process of T7   opposite the inferior angle of the scapulae.

For locating spinous processes use the **Rule of Threes**:-

T1-3	spinous process is at the same level as own transverse process.
T4-6	spinous process is at the level between own and next transverse process.
T7-9	spinous process is at the level over transverse process of next vertebrae.

The spinous process of T8 is the longest and may just overlap the superior border of T10.

T10-12	T12 is like T1; T11 is like T5; T10 is like T9.

Positions and patterns

Resting	midway between flexion and extension
Close packed	extension

Active range of movement

flexion	20-45°	**rotation**	35-50°
extension	25-45°	**side-bending**	20-40°

Movement of the ribs

The movement of the ribs at the costovertebral joints is described as pump handle in the upper rib cage and bucket handle in the lower ribs. The type of movement is determined by the angle of the transverse process to the vertebral body and the angle made by the neck of the rib and the body at the tubercle.

In the upper ribs, the axis from the articulation on the vertebral body to the tip of the transverse process is almost in the coronal plane. This axis causes the movement at the joint complex to create an increase in the anterior-posterior diameter of the thorax - the pump handle movement.

In the lower ribs, the axis from the articulation on the vertebral body to the tip of the transverse process is almost sagittal. This axis causes the movement at the joint complex to create an increase in the lateral diameter of the thorax - the bucket handle movement.

The general respiratory mechanics will vary with age, sex and position. It is said that in the erect position:-

♦ women primarily use the upper thoracic complex for relaxed breathing;
♦ men use both the upper and lower thoracic complex for relaxed breathing;
♦ children primarily use the lower thoracic complex for relaxed breathing.

When sitting or lying supine, the abdominal contents push the diaphragm upward so reducing the range of movement available for inspiration.

In the side-lying position, the abdominal contents push upward on to the lower aspect of the diaphragm thus reducing movement which is restricted by the pressure of the body on the ribs.

With age, the increasing kyphosis, reduced tone of the abdominal muscles and loss of elasticity of the costal cartilage increase low thoracic and abdominal breathing in both sexes.

Hands on: a clinical companion

Special tests for the thoracic spine and ribs

Impingement tests

Slump test / dural stretch
The elements are added in the following order. Once nerve pain is reproduced the test is considered positive and concluded. The test begins with the patient sitting slumped upon the treatment table looking straight ahead with their legs over the edge and knees at 90° flexion. If this position causes no pain the practitioner flexes the patient's neck, extends one knee, and finally dorsiflexes the foot of the straight leg. The test is repeated on the other leg.

Other tests

T1 nerve root
The patient sits on the treatment table and actively abducts the shoulder to 90° with the forearm pronated and elbow flexed to 90°. There should be **NO** pain. The patient then fully flexes the elbow and places their hand behind their head. The ulnar nerve and T1 nerve root are stretched in this position and pain in the T1 distribution is a positive test.

Winging of scapulae
The patient stands facing a wall with arms flexed to 90° pushing onto the wall. A positive sign is where one scapula appears to project posteriorly off the rib cage, indicating there is a lesion within the long thoracic nerve causing weakness or paralysis of the serratus anterior muscle on that side.

Chest expansion
The chest circumference, at a named specific level, is measured at full expiration and again at the point of maximum inspiration. The difference in the two measurements is the chest expansion and this should normally be between 5-10cm.

Chapter 6

The lumbar spine

This area of the spine is designed for strength, stability and mobility. The lumbar vertebrae [Figure 6.1] reflect this and are particularly large and heavy. The body is wider transversely and slightly kidney-shaped. The lower three are slightly wedged, higher anteriorly than posteriorly, which enhances the normal lordosis. The pedicles are short and arise from the upper part of the body, the superior vertebral notch is small and the inferior notch is much deeper.

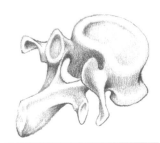

Figure 6.1 A typical lumbar vertebra.

The transverse process projects laterally and slightly posteriorly, the distal part represents a rudimentary fused rib. On the base is a small tubercle, the accessory process that is dwarfed by the larger mammillary process on the superior articular process. The lamina are shorter vertically than elsewhere in the spine and in the midline unite and form the spinous process. This is broad and narrow with an enlarged tip.

Ligaments of the lumbar spine

Anterior ligaments

Anterior longitudinal ligament
The anterior longitudinal ligament is firmly attached to the body and discs.

Posterior ligaments

Supraspinous ligament
This runs over the tips of the spinous processes and blends with the strong interspinous ligaments that join adjacent spinous processes.

Ligamentum flavum

A paired flat ligament that runs between adjacent laminae, and blends with the joint capsule.

Posterior longitudinal ligament

Narrow over the body, expanding over the ends of the bodies and intervening disc. It is firmly attached to the ends of the bodies and discs, but is separated from the bodies by connective tissue that contains the blood vessels to and from the bone.

Transverse ligament

This runs between the accessory tubercles on adjacent transverse processes.

Iliolumbar ligament [Figure 6.2]

Divided into two bands, the superior and the inferior. The superior band runs from the tip of the transverse process of L4 laterally, inferiorly and posteriorly to its insertion on the iliac crest. The inferior band runs from the tip of the transverse process of L5 laterally and inferiorly to its insertion on the iliac crest slightly anterior to the superior band and to the anterior surface of the sacrum.

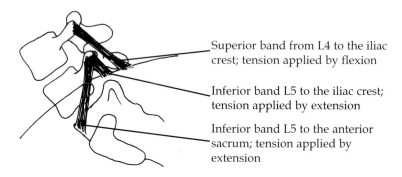

Superior band from L4 to the iliac crest; tension applied by flexion

Inferior band L5 to the iliac crest; tension applied by extension

Inferior band L5 to the anterior sacrum; tension applied by extension

Figure 6.2 Iliolumbar ligament.

In active movements the superior band acts to limit flexion of L4 and L5. The inferior band, due to the direction of the fibres, will limit extension of the lumbosacral segment.

Intervertebral disc

These are between all the vertebral bodies, except the atlas and axis. Each disc comprises a central gelatinous part, the nucleus pulposus situated slightly within the posterior portion of the disc and a fibrous covering, the annulus fibrosus. The fibres of the annulus are arranged in concentric circles, like the layers of an onion. However, each layer has a different slant to the preceding one, increasing the strength of the structure without limiting its flexibility. Signs of degeneration are apparent from the third decade and result in microcracks forming between the layers weakening the whole structure.

Muscles of the lumbar spine

Muscles acting upon the lumbar spine can be divided two groups, those directly related to and those unrelated to the vertebral column. The muscles unrelated to the vertebral column are listed in Table 4. The muscles directly related to the vertebral column can be further subdivided into superficial, intermediate [Table 1] and deep [Tables 2 and 3].

Table 1 The superficial and intermediate muscles of the lumbar spine.

Superficial layer		
	Origin	Insertion
Latissimus dorsi	S/P T7-L5, sacrum, iliac crest	Floor of bicipital groove
Intermediate layer		
Serratus posterior inferior	S/P T11-L2	Posterior ribs 9-12
Quadratus lumborum	12th rib T/P L1-4	T/P L1-4, iliac crest
Psoas	T/P L1-4, anterior vertebral bodies, discs	Lesser trochanter of femur

The deep muscles of the spine are the erector spinae, transversospinalis and the segmental muscles. The segmental muscles are the deepest layer consisting of short and long rotators and the interspinalis group passing between adjoining vertebral spinous processes.

Erector spinae

This group of muscles makes up the largest muscle bulk in the back. There is a common origin from the sacrum, iliac crest and spinous processes of most of the lumbar vertebrae. The muscle divides into three vertical columns: the iliocostalis [lateral], the longissimus [intermediate] and the spinalis [medial].

Each muscle is named after the spinal area in which it is found. However, the spinalis is generally poorly defined and blends with longissimus thoracis in the thorax and semispinalis capitis in the neck.

Table 2 The erector spinae muscle of the lumbar spine.

		Origin	Insertion
Iliocostalis	lumborum	Iliac crest and sacrum, S/Ps lumbar spine	Near angles of lower 6-7 ribs
	thoracis	Upper borders of lower 6-7 ribs	Near angles of upper 6-7 ribs
	cervicis	Upper borders of upper 6-7 ribs	T/P C4-6
Longissimus	thoracis	Sacrum, S/P T8-L5	Lower 9-10 ribs and associated T/Ps
	cervicis	T/P T1-6	T/P C2-6
	capitis	Articular pillars C4-7	Mastoid process
Spinalis		S/Ps at lower vertebral levels	All S/Ps, base of skull

Transversospinalis and interspinalis muscles

This group is comprised of three muscles: the semispinalis, the multifidus and the rotators. The muscles are short generally from one vertebrae to the next or one above. Interspinalis muscles pass from the superior border of one spinous process inserting in the inferior border of the spinous process immediately above.

Table 3 The transversospinalis and interspinalis muscles.

		Origin	**Insertion**
Semispinalis	thoracis	T/P T6-12	S/P T1-6, C5-7
	cervicis	T/P T1-6	S/P C2-T5
	capitis	T/P T1-6, articular processes C4-6	Between nuchal lines on occiput
Multifidus	lumborum	Sacrum and mamillary processes	S/P above origin
	thoracis	T/Ps	S/P above origin
	cervicis	T/Ps	S/P above origin
Rotators		Deepest on T/Ps	S/P next vertebrae or one above
Interspinalis		S/P superior border	S/P inferior border

Active movements of the trunk and lumbar spine

The main muscles involved in moving the trunk and lumbar spine when the hips and pelvis are fixed are listed in Table 5. In flexion or extension, the muscles act on both sides equally. When the movement is side-bending, the ipsilateral muscles act but rotation is achieved by a combination of ipsilateral and contralateral muscles. Psoas, due to its origin on the anterior aspect of the vertebral column, will assist in flexion of the whole trunk. If its action is limited to the lumbar spine, it will assist in extension.

Table 4 Muscles of the abdomen and trunk offering support to the vertebral column.

Abdomen and trunk		
	Origin	Insertion
Rectus abdominis	Crest and symphysis of pubis	Costal cartilages R5- 7
External oblique	Angles of lower 8 ribs	Iliac crest, pubis
Internal oblique	Rectus sheath, costal margin	Lumbar fascia, iliac crest
Transverse abdominis	Costal margin, lumbar fascia, iliac crest	Rectus abdominis sheath
Quadratus lumborum	12th rib T/P L1-4	T/P L1-4, iliac crest

Table 5 The main muscles for movement in the trunk and lumbar spine when the hips and pelvis are fixed.

Movement	Bilateral or ipsilateral muscle action	Contralateral muscle action
Flexion	Rectus abdominis, external oblique, internal oblique, psoas [trunk only]	
Extension	Erector spinae, latissimus dorsi, trapezius, serratus posterior inferior, quadratus lumborum, psoas [lumbar spine only]	
Side-bending	Quadratus lumborum, internal oblique, external oblique, psoas, latissimus dorsi, serratus posterior inferior, trapezius, erector spinae [ipsilateral]	
Rotation	Internal oblique, latissimus dorsi, serratus posterior inferior, short and long rotators	External oblique, psoas

Differential diagnosis in the lumbar spine

Tables 6 and 7 are not designed to be the means to a definite diagnosis for the commonest lumbar musculoskeletal problems but identify the commonest and classical symptoms associated with each condition. It is important to remember that every patient is unique; how they react to and interpret their symptoms provides the practitioner with the challenge of making a diagnosis.

Table 6 covers the common conditions that tend to be associated with the younger patient. These conditions usually have a sudden onset and an acute pattern. However, they can become recurrent and develop into chronic conditions.

Table 6 Conditions associated with a younger patient.

	Herniated disc	Spondylolisthesis	Facet irritation
Age at onset [yrs]	18-45	20-40	20-50
Pain site	Low back, nerve pain referral	Central low back	Localised sharp
Onset	Acute or following previous episodes	Insidious	Acute sudden
Aggravated by	Sitting, coughing, sneezing, pressure on low back	Prolonged standing or unsupported sitting, repetitive bending	Specific movements, facet compression
Relieved by	Standing, protective posture, lying, bending	Rest, sitting supported	Static posture
Special tests	Valsalva, straight leg raise, compression	Palpable step, x-ray	Compression, straight leg raise

Spondylolisthesis is the term applied to the condition of spondylolysis once slippage of the vertebral body has occurred.

Conditions associated with the more mature patient [Table 7] are usually degenerative in nature and tend to have an insidious onset and develop a chronic recurrent pattern.

Table 7 Conditions associated with the mature patient.

	Osteoarthrosis	Spinal stenosis	Ligament strain
Age at onset [yrs]	Over 50	Over 60	Over 40
Pain site	Generalised	Bilateral to legs	Vague, deep in low back
Onset	Insidious	Insidious	Insidious or sudden
Aggravated by	Prolonged standing, difficulty getting out of chair, stiff in the mornings	Extension, standing, possibly lying supine	Prolonged standing or sitting, slow walking, wearing heels
Relieved by	Support while sitting, lying, gentle activity	Sitting, bending, rest	Fast walking, gentle mobility, lying on side
Special tests	X ray	X-ray, straight leg raise	

Common pathological conditions of the lumbar spine

Deformities

Scoliosis
Any lateral plane curvature of the spine, no matter the cause. This can be divided into protective, functional or structural. Protective or functional are temporary and can be due to pain or short-term posture. When structural changes occur the scoliosis becomes permanent. This can be due to a short leg [actual or functional], hemivertebra or abnormal vertebrae [congenital or traumatic], or muscle weakness.

Lordosis
This is defined as any increase in the normal curve in the lumbar spine. It can be divided into two types:-

Functional or temporary
This can be seen in any lumbar spine, during pregnancy, whilst carrying heavy loads or after prolonged standing. The normal lordosis will return at the end of the activity or after a period of rest.

Permanent
When structural changes have occurred either due to a congenital abnormality, prolonged persistent poor posture, poor muscular strength or a large protruding abdomen. A return to the normal lordosis is not possible.

Spina bifida
Variable degree of deformity from a split spinous process to a wide defect in the neural arch.

Spondylolysis
This can either be congenital or traumatic. When slippage occurs, it is called spondylolisthesis. Symptoms include chronic aching, recurrent bouts of pain aggravated by standing. X-rays will show the defect in pars interarticularis. There is a palpable step between the spinous processes at the level above where the slippage has occurred.

Spinal stenosis
Often seen in the 60+ age group and associated with osteoarthritic changes and bilateral symptoms in the legs. An insidious onset which may eventually affect bladder and bowel control.

Osteoporosis
Commonest within the thoracic spine but can ocur in the lumbar spine. It will generally occur if there is a prolonged period of confinement to bed, and in association with parathyroid osteodystrophy or Cushing's syndrome. Percussion is occasionally tender on the spinous processes and spontaneous unexplained fractures can occur leading to sudden reduction in height.

Scheuermann's disease
This affects children between 13-16 years of age, especially in the thoracic spine. In the lumbar spine it only affects one or two vertebra. The

condition affects the development of cartilage end plates and ring epiphyses causing localised pain and herniation of disc material into the vertebral body. The affected segment has reduced mobility and is slightly deformed, reducing the normal lordosis and mobility in the area.

Infections

Pyogenic
This is uncommon. The spread occurs via the vascular system either by blood or lymph. The patient has a temperature and another site of infection.

Tuberculosis
The foci is in the anterior margin of the vertebral body commonly in young adults. It is the commonest site with the thoracic spine for tuberculosis, often leading to the involvement of psoas and an abscess in the groin. The patient looks ill; there is local tenderness on firm palpation/percussion, with protective muscle spasm, a protective posture, stiffness and swelling. The spinal cord can be involved.

Arthritis

Rheumatoid arthritis
Occasionally this affects the lumbar spine, but there will be symptoms from other joints. If affected, the spine will be stiff and swollen with reduction in all ranges of movement.

Osteoarthritis
Very common in the low lumbar spine especially in the elderly patient. In younger patients, symptoms occur in 30% of patients who have x-ray signs of spondylosis.

Ankylosing spondylitis
This gradually spreads up from the pelvis and initially will cause a reduction in the lordosis and both active and passive range of movements. Eventually fusion of the spine occurs with a characteristic bamboo spine on x-ray.

Polymyalgia rheumatica
Occurs especially in the 60+ age group, women three times as often as men. The patient presents with morning stiffness across the pelvis and low back that lasts for at least one hour. In the day the symptoms can return to normal with little stiffness or pain. A raised ESR is indicative, and corticosteroid therapy will clear the symptoms almost immediately. The condition will last for between 2-4 years requiring progressively less medication to control the symptoms. A patient can occasionally have similar symptoms in the shoulder girdle.

Paget's disease
Dull aching pain aggravated by use or immobility, affecting men twice more often than women in the 40+ age group. Of unknown aetiology, it affects, in particular the pelvis, femur, skull, tibia and vertebrae.

Mechanical

Prolapsed disc
Commonest in the 18-45 age range, with a recent history of trauma involving lifting. Sharp, localised pain with referred pain and paraesthesia to the lower limb following a dermatomal pattern.

Tumours

In all cases the collapse of bone will involve the nerve.

Bone
Metastatic carcinoma.

Cord
Neurofibroma.

Nerve
Neurofibroma.

Common extrinsic causes of symptoms

These are generally due to serious pathological conditions. The symptom picture will be:-

♦ an insidious onset, progressively increasing symptoms that are not relieved by rest, and unremitting night pain;
♦ symptoms are generalised and linked to multiple spinal levels;
♦ associated pain in the thoracic spine;
♦ a generalised systemic illness, unexpected weight loss or prolonged steroid use.

Urinary system

Renal conditions, prostatic cancer or hypertrophy, testicular cancer.

Cardiovascular system

Abdominal aortic aneurysm, endocarditis.

Gastrointestinal system

Obstruction of intestines, Crohn's disease, ulcerative colitis.

Gynaecological

Endometriosis, salpingitis or dysmenorrhoea, ectopic or normal pregnancy, ovarian cyst or fibroids.

Although these constitute red flag conditions that require referral, the following symptoms indicate the presence of a condition that requires **immediate referral** for emergency investigation and surgical treatment:-

♦ loss of bladder or bowel control;
♦ saddle area sensory disturbance or loss of sphincter control;
♦ total sensory loss on neurological examination;
♦ bilateral leg pain with bilateral neurological deficit.

Physical examination of the lumbar spine

The main bony landmark of the lumbar spine is the lumbosacral junction. This can be found in several ways:-

♦ palpate the upper limit of the posterior superior iliac spine, bisect the two points and this will be over L5;
♦ palpate the sulcus under the posterior superior iliac spine [at S2], count the spinous processes up to L5;
♦ palpate the most superior point of the iliac crest, bisect these two points to find L4, count the spinous processes down to L5.

Positions and patterns

Resting	midway between flexion and extension
Close packed	extension

Active range of movement

flexion	40-60°	**rotation**	3-18°
extension	20-35°	**side-bending**	15-20°

The lumbar vertebral discs undergo a wide variety of pressure changes during normal activities. The following list illustrates how much the pressure changes within the disc of L3 as a percentage of the pressure exerted when standing relaxed and erect.

♦ Sitting leaning forward	275%
♦ Bending to 45° [legs straight]	200%
♦ Standing up from a chair	175%
♦ Bending to 80° [legs straight]	150%
♦ Sitting upright, no support	150%
♦ Standing erect	100%
♦ Lying prone	75%
♦ Lying supine	25%

Special tests for the lumbar spine

Impingement tests

Slump test/dural stretch

The elements are added in the following order. Once nerve pain is reproduced, the test is considered positive and is concluded. The test begins with the patient sitting slumped upon the treatment table looking straight ahead with their legs over the edge and knees at 90° flexion. If this position causes no pain, the practitioner flexes the patient's neck, extends one knee, and finally dorsiflexes the foot of the straight leg. The test is repeated on the other leg. A positive test indicates a spinal cord, nerve root or sciatic nerve impingement. The test can be modified for the obturator nerve by abducting the hip before extending the knee and dorsiflexing the foot.

Nerve stretch tests

Straight leg raise test, also known as Lasague's test

The patient lies supine. The pain-free leg is tested first. The practitioner places the hip in slight medial rotation and adduction before slowly lifting the straight leg from the ankle, ensuring the quadriceps remain relaxed. Once pain is felt in the back or posterior thigh, the hip flexion is slightly reduced, to clear the pain, and passive dorsiflexion of the foot applied. If pain occurs the test is positive. If there is no pain, the patient is asked to actively fully flex their neck.

In the above, the neck flexion has also been called Hyndman's sign, Brudzinski's sign or Lindner's sign. The ankle dorsiflexion movement is also known as Braggard's test. Pain that increases with either neck flexion or ankle dorsiflexion or both, indicates stretching of the dura mater of the spinal cord. Possible causes include disc herniation, a tumour or meningitis. Pain that does not increase with neck flexion may indicate a lesion in the hamstrings, lumbosacral or sacroiliac regions.

The test can be modified to stress different peripheral nerves as noted in Table 8.

Table 8 Modifications to the basic straight leg raise test.

	Straight leg raise basic	Tibial nerve	Sural nerve	Common peroneal nerve
Hip	Flexion, slight medial rotation and adduction	Flexion	Flexion	Flexion, medial rotation
Knee	Extension		Extension	
Ankle	Dorsiflexion			Plantar flexion
Foot		Eversion	Inversion	Inversion
Toes		Extension		

Femoral nerve L2/3/4 traction test

The patient lies on the unaffected side with the low back in the easy normal position and slight flexion induced into the cervical spine. The unaffected lower leg is flexed at the hip and knee for stability. The practitioner grasps the upper leg, keeping the thigh parallel to the table, and passively extends the knee while applying 15° of extension to the hip. The knee is then carefully flexed until pain radiates into the anterior thigh. This is considered a positive test.

Nachlas test femoral nerve L2/3/4

The patient lies prone with the cervical spine rotated to the test side and the rest of the spine in a relaxed neutral position. The practitioner passively fully flexes the knee, ensuring that the hip remains in the midline with no rotation. If this flexion is limited to under 90° by knee pathology the hip should be extended. A positive test causes pain in the buttock or leg indicating a L2 or L3 nerve root lesion. Pain can be due to tight quadriceps, or sacroiliac torsion.

The test can be modified to stress different peripheral nerves. By adding adduction and extension of the hip to the basic test, the lateral femoral nerve is stretched.

If the hip is abducted, extended and laterally rotated, while extending the knee, dorsiflexing the ankle and everting the foot, the saphenous nerve is stretched.

Compression tests

Active compression test [Valsalva]

The seated patient is asked to take a breath, hold and bear down as if evacuating the bowels. An increase in pain indicates a positive test.

Passive compression test

The practitioner stands behind the sitting patient to support and apply a graded pressure through the shoulder girdle to compress the lumbar spine. Initially, compression is applied through the erect spine followed by compression in flexion, extension, side-bending and the intermediate quadrants.

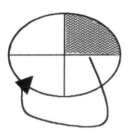

An increase in symptoms following compression of the spine in the quadrant indicated, [flexion combined with side-bending away from the symptomatic side], combined with no increase in symptoms following compression in extension and side-bending towards the symptomatic side, suggests a disc herniation.

[The arrow indicates the recommended path to follow when moving from compression in flexion to extension and side-bending when a disc herniation is suspected.]

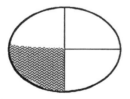

An increase in symptoms following compression of the spine in the quadrant indicated, [extension combined with side-bending towards the symptomatic side] indicates a foraminal impingement or facet problem.

Figure 6.3 Compression tests showing the possible pattern for a disc herniation and nerve root entrapment.

Chapter 7

The pelvis

The bony pelvis [Figure 7.1], differs between the sexes. The male is longer and narrower with the sacral base approximately a third of the breadth; the female is broader with a wider pelvic brim. The pelvic bowl comprises three paired bones: the ilium, the pubis and the ischium that unite forming the acetabulum and the unpaired sacrum and coccyx. The iliac bones articulate with the sacrum at the sacroiliac joint posteriorly and the pubic bones at the symphysis pubis anteriorly.

Ilium	The largest bone forms the upper part of the acetabulum and shape of pelvis superiorly.
Pubis	The body forms the symphysis pubis and passes posteriorly dividing into two rami, superior and inferior. These border the obturator foramen before joining the ischium, the inferior at the ischial tuberosity and the superior in the acetabulum.
Ischium	The body forms part of the acetabulum and the rami bound the inferior aspect of the obturator foramen ending at the ischial tuberosity.

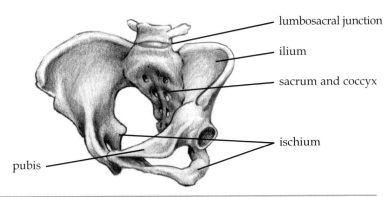

Figure 7.1 The bony pelvis.

The sacrum is a triangular bone formed by fusion of the five sacral vertebrae. The pelvic surface is smooth whilst the dorsal surface has crests and ridges. The median crest replaces the spinous processes, the intermediate forms the articular processes, and the lateral crest is the fused transverse and costal process.

There are paired foramen for the spinal nerves, on the pelvic surface for the ventral branches and on the dorsal surface for the dorsal branches.

The coccyx represents the final four vertebrae of the spinal column, and are generally fused together. The first articulates with the sacrum with a rudimentary disc.

The sacroiliac joint is a plane synovial joint between the sacrum and the ilium. The many irregular elevations and depressions on the articular surface increase with age and develop to resist the shearing movement, so adding strength to the joint whilst transferring load. The joint is a crescent shape and is lined by hyaline cartilage on the ilium that is three times thicker than the fibrocartilage on the sacrum. On the sacral surface of the joint at the junction between the longer cranial and caudal segment is a regular depression. A corresponding elevation on the iliac surface causes the joint to rotate around this point. The normal range of movement varies but is generally very small. With age, fibrous or fibrocartilaginous adhesions reduce the mobility of the joint to the point, particularly in men, of total fusion.

The symphysis pubis is a secondary cartilaginous joint with minimal mobility situated on the anterior margin of the pelvis. It is lined by hyaline cartilage and joined by a fibrocartilaginous disc with a small central cleft.

The pelvis as a unit will transmit the weight of the body equally to the legs, form a stable bony base to the abdominal cavity and provide attachment points for muscles to aid an upright stance. It also fixes the inferior end of the spinal cord and provides a wide base on which to sit. The sacroiliac joint and the symphysis pubis give the pelvis elasticity and assist in absorbing and dissipating the forces of walking and running.

Ligaments of the pelvis [Figure 7.2]

As one of the main functions of the pelvis is to transmit the body's weight to the legs, the pelvic ligaments must be very strong to limit the natural movements of the sacroiliac joint.

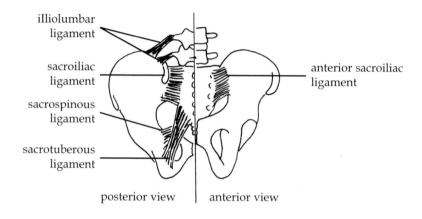

Figure 7.2 Ligaments of the sacroiliac joint and pelvis.

Table 1 The posterior and anterior ligaments of the pelvis.

Posterior ligaments

	Plane of ligament	Origin/insertion
Iliolumbar	Superior	T/P L4 to iliac crest
	Inferior	T/P L5, iliac crest and anterior-superior surface of sacrum
Sacroiliac	Intermediate plane	Iliac crest to transverse tubercle of S1
		Iliac crest to the other sacral tubercles
	Anterior plane	Posterior iliac crest to articular tubercles
Sacrospinous		Ischial spine to border sacrum and coccyx
Sacrotuberous		Ischial tuberosity to ilium, sacrum and coccyx

Anterior ligaments

Sacroiliac	Superior	Ilium to S1
	Inferior	Ilium to the other sacral segments

The sacrotuberous and sacrospinous ligaments divide the sciatic notch into two: a superior or greater notch for piriformis and an inferior or lesser notch for obturator internus. There are also three sets of ligaments not shown in the diagrams: the axial or interosseous sacroiliac, the sacrococcygeal ligaments and those associated with the symphysis pubis.

Axial or interosseous sacroiliac ligament

These are deep to the posterior sacroiliac ligament and lie on the axis of rotation of the sacroiliac joint, keeping it in close approximation.

Sacrococcygeal ligaments

These ligaments act to reduce the movements between the sacrum and coccyx.

Anterior sacrococcygeal
This runs from the anterior surface of the sacrum to the coccyx.

Lateral sacrococcygeal
This runs from the lateral aspect of the sacrum to the coccyx.

Posterior sacrococcygeal
This runs from the posterior surface of the sacrum to the coccyx.

Ligaments of the symphysis pubis

The anterior aspect of the symphysis pubis is supported and strengthened by the anterior ligament and an aponeurotic expansion from the rectus abdominis, transversus, adductor longus and pyramidalis.

The posterior, superior and inferior ligaments pass between the pubic bones and add strength to the symphysis.

Muscles of the pelvis

The sacroiliac joint is one of the few joints in the body that has no muscles acting directly over it. The muscles that affect the sacroiliac joint and the pelvis can be grouped into four general functional groups, identified by letters A-D in Figure 7.3 below:-

A lumbar erector spinae, spinal extensors.
B biceps femoris, adductors.
C iliopsoas, rectus femoris.
D rectus abdominis, other abdominal muscles.

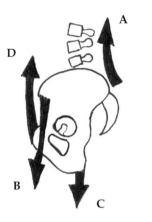

Stability of the pelvis in the lateral plane with the weight equally transmitted through both legs is achieved by simultaneous contraction of the ipsilateral and contralateral adductors and abductors. If contractions are not balanced, the pelvis will tilt towards the side of adductor predominance. When standing on one leg, the stability comes from the contraction of ipsilateral abductors only.

Figure 7.3 Lateral view of the muscles of the pelvis.

In the posterior plane with the hips extended, the centre of gravity is slightly behind the transverse axis of the hips. Balance is maintained by tension in the hip ligaments and tensor fasciae latae. With the pelvis slightly tilted posteriorly, gluteus minimus helps keep balance and when the trunk flexes, the muscles contract in turn: gluteus maximus, then piriformis, obturator internus and quadratus femoris.

Hands on: a clinical companion

Muscles that specifically have an effect are shown in Figures 7.4 and 7.5 and briefly described in Table 2.

Table 2 Muscles affecting the pelvis.

Anterior view [Figure 7.4]

	Origin	Insertion
Psoas	T/P L1-4, anterior vertebral bodies, discs	Lesser trochanter of femur
Iliacus	Inner surface iliac fossa	Lesser trochanter of femur
External oblique	Lower 8 ribs	Iliac crest, pubis
Internal oblique	Rectus sheath, costal margin	Lumbar fascia, iliac crest
Rectus abdominis	Pubic crest and symphysis	Costal cartilages ribs 5-7

Posterior view [Figure 7.5]

Quadratus lumborum	12th rib T/P L1-4	T/P L1-4, iliac crest
Gluteus maximus	Rim of ilium, sacrum, coccyx	Iliotibial tract
Gluteus medius	Outer aspect of ilium	Greater trochanter
Gluteus minimus	Outer aspect of ilium	Greater trochanter
Piriformis	Pelvic surface sacrum	Greater trochanter
Gemellus superior/inferior	Ischial spine, ilium	Greater trochanter
Obturator internus/ externus	Obturator foramen	Greater trochanter

Not shown in Figure 7.5 but affecting the pelvis

Latissimus dorsi	S/P T7-L5, sacrum, iliac crest	Floor of bicipital groove

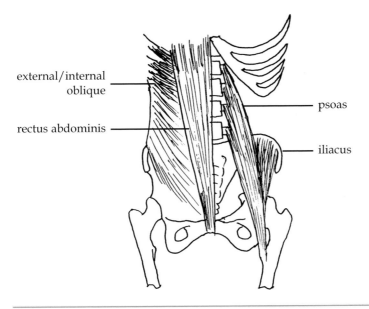

Figure 7.4 Anterior view of the muscles of the pelvis.

external/internal oblique

rectus abdominis

psoas

iliacus

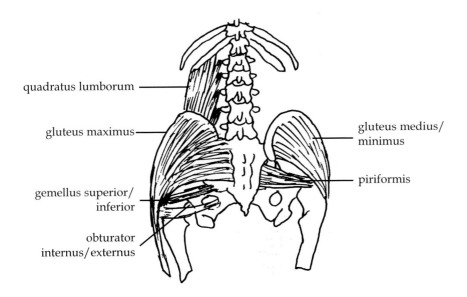

quadratus lumborum

gluteus maximus

gemellus superior/ inferior

obturator internus/externus

gluteus medius/ minimus

piriformis

Figure 7.5 Posterior view of the muscles of the pelvis.

Common pathological conditions of the pelvis

Arthritis

Ankylosing spondylitis
A chronic condition of the sacroiliac joints and spine leading to a progressive calcification of the spinal ligaments affecting men five times more than women. The onset is between 15-30 years of age and can eventually affect the hips or peripheral joints. The patient presents with bilateral pain, prolonged morning stiffness for over one hour and can have iritis and aortic incompetence. Active movements are grossly reduced. The patient is unable to sit with their legs straight without support. There are no passive movements possible in the sacroiliac joint. X-rays show ankylosis, the ESR is raised and the antigen HLA-B27 is present in blood tests.

Polymyalgia rheumatica
Especially in the 60+ age group, occuring in women three times as often as men. Occasionally, a patient can have similar symptoms in the shoulder girdle. The patient presents with bilateral pain and morning stiffness that lasts for at least one hour. The onset can be sudden and the symptoms can return to normal with little stiffness or pain during the day. A raised ESR is indicative, and corticosteroid therapy will clear the symptoms almost immediately. The condition will last for between 2-4 years requiring progressively less medication to control the symptoms.

Paget's disease
Dull aching pain aggravated by use or immobility, affecting men twice more often than women in the 40+ age group. Of unknown aetiology, it affects, in particular the pelvis, femur, skull, tibia and vertebrae.

Others

Any condition in the lumbar spine can refer to the pelvis including any of the pathological conditions previously listed. Specifically, conditions that may cause symptoms include:-

♦ vascular occlusion, inguinal hernia, pressure over the femoral triangle from a large abdomen;

- gynaecological conditions such as endometriosis, salpingitis or dysmenorrhoea;
- intra-pelvic mass, such as an ectopic or normal pregnancy, ovarian cyst or fibroids;
- osteoarthritis of the hip;
- diseases of the large bowel including Crohn's disease.

Physical examination of the pelvis

When examining the sacroiliac joint, a subjective finding of no movement, or x-rays that show ankylosis can be normal particularly in middle-aged or older men.

The main bony landmarks of the pelvis are superiorly, the iliac crest; anteriorly, the anterior superior iliac spine [ASIS]; and posteriorly, the posterior superior iliac spine [PSIS].

These landmarks can be palpated by first finding the iliac crest, the most superior part of the bony pelvis:-

To palpate the ASIS	From the iliac crest, follow this bone anteriorly until a sulcus is felt. This is just inferior to the ASIS.
To palpate the PSIS	From the iliac crest, follow this bone posteriorly until a sulcus is felt. This is just inferior to the PSIS.

Positions and patterns

Resting	neutral
Capsular pattern	pain when joint stressed

As mentioned before, there are no muscles acting directly over the sacroiliac joint, so movement is induced by tissue tension following movement in the adjacent areas. The approximate ranges of motion normally needed in these adjacent joints before the sacroiliac joint is stressed are listed below:-

Movement of the spine		Movement of the hip			
flexion	45°	flexion	110°	extension	10°
extension	25°	abduction	40°	adduction	30°
rotation	5°	medial rotation	35°	lateral rotation	40°
side-bending	15°				

Movement of the pelvis

There are many different theories about how the pelvis moves and how that movement should be described. The following is the nutation and counternutation theory. In Latin *nutare* means to nod and in this description of the movement of the pelvis refers to the movement of the sacral base.

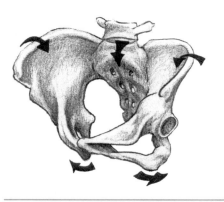

The sacroiliac joint moves around its axis of rotation allowing the sacral base to move anteriorly and the coccyx posteriorly.

The movement of the sacrum causes the two ischial tuberosities to move slightly outwards, the iliac crest slightly inwards and the iliac bones to rotate posteriorly.

Figure 7.6 Nutation of the pelvis.

In the erect position, the sacroiliac joint will naturally nutate due to the weight of the trunk being transmitted through the lordotic lumbar spine. The strong iliolumbar, sacrospinous, sacrotuberous and anterior sacro-iliac ligaments resist this movement.

During the opposite movement of counternutation, the sacral base moves posteriorly, the coccyx anteriorly, the ischial tuberosities slightly inwards, the iliac crest outwards and the iliac bone rotates anteriorly. This movement of counternutation is resisted solely by the sacroiliac ligaments.

Special tests for the pelvis

Stress tests [active] for the sacroiliac joint

Standing tests

Flamingo test
The patient stands and flexes one knee with the foot on the ground, resulting in all their weight being carried by one leg. This causes the sacrum to move forward and stresses the weight-bearing joint. Pain indicates a positive test.

Gillet's test / Stork test
While the patient stands, the practitioner palpates the spinous process of S2 and one PSIS. The patient is then asked to stand on the opposite leg, supporting themselves with one hand whilst flexing the non weight-bearing hip to at least 90° [the non-supporting hand can assist this hip flexion]. The test is repeated with the other leg. Normal movement through the sacroiliac joint will result either in no relative movement between the PSIS and S2 or a slight inferior movement of the PSIS relative to the S2 spinous process. If the sacroiliac joint is restricted, the relative movement of the PSIS on that side will be in a superior direction.

Kinetic flexion test / Standing flexion test
While the patient stands, the practitioner palpates the PSISs. The relative positions of the PSISs are noted and the patient is asked to flex the trunk forward. At the limit of flexion, the new relative positions are noted, and the patient asked to stand upright again. In a normal pelvis both PSISs would move equally in a superior and anterior direction. If one PSIS moves first and moves further cephalically, it indicates either that this sacroiliac joint is restricted or the other has been prevented from moving.

Sitting tests

Seated flexion test
This test follows the kinetic flexion test with the patient sitting on the treatment table with their feet flat on the floor. The practitioner palpates the PSISs, noting their relative positions and the patient is asked to flex the trunk with their hands between their knees. At the limit of flexion, the new relative positions are noted, and the patient asked to return to an upright

sitting position. The test is considered positive if one PSIS moves more cephalically than the other.

If the findings correspond to the standing test results - one PSIS moves first and further cephalically - this indicates that the sacroiliac joint is restricted. If the results differ from the standing test, it will indicate one of the following:-

♦ a reduction in relative movement of the PSIS indicates an iliosacral problem, the restriction being caused by tight hamstrings or glutei;
♦ an increase in relative movement of the PSIS indicates increased tone in the quadratus lumborum or erector spinae or the problem is in the lumbar spine.

Sit to supine test

The patient sits on the treatment table with both their legs straight.

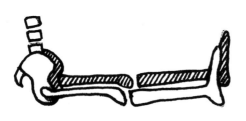

The relative positions of the medial malleoli are palpated and noted.

It can be seen that the medial malleolus on the shaded side is lower than the non-shaded side.

The patient is then asked to lie on the treatment table with both their legs straight.

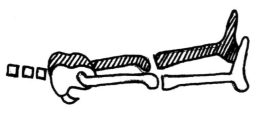

The relative positions of the medial malleoli are again palpated and noted.

It can be seen that the medial malleolus on the shaded side is now held higher than the non-shaded side.

Figure 7.7 The sit to supine test.

The following assumptions can be made from these relative positions:-

- ◆ if the innominate is held posteriorly rotated, that medial malleolus will be lower when the patient is sitting but higher than the other when the patient is lying supine [dark shaded leg, Figure 7.7];
- ◆ if the innominate is held anteriorly rotated, that medial malleolus will be higher when the patient is sitting but lower than the other when lying supine [non-shaded leg, Figure 7.7].

Stress tests [passive] for the sacroiliac joint

Passive lateral rotation of the hip
This should only be conducted if the hip has a normal range of movement. The patient lies supine on the treatment table, with one hip and knee flexed to 90°. The hip is passively laterally rotated to its limit placing stress upon the sacroiliac joint.

Sacroiliac knee to shoulder
The patient lies supine and the practitioner passively flexes the knee and hip whilst adducting and medially rotating the hip. Direct pressure down the shaft of the femur will stress the sacrotuberous ligament.

Gapping test - supine
The patient lies supine and the practitioner crosses their hands over the patient's pelvis to cup both the ASISs. An outward pressure on the ASIS stresses the anterior structures of the sacroiliac joints. Pain indicates a positive test.

Squish test - supine
The patient lies supine and the practitioner places each hand on the outer aspect of the ASIS. The practitioner compresses the ASISs together stressing the posterior structures of the sacroiliac joints. Pain indicates a positive test.

Chapter 8

The shoulder complex

This is a complex functional group comprising of four joints, three synovial and one muscular, three bones and at least 17 separate muscles.

The three bones involved are the scapula, humerus and clavicle. The synovial joints are the glenohumeral, acromioclavicular and sternoclavicular and the muscular joint is between the thoracic cage and the scapula creating the scapulothoracic joint. Although not a true joint, movement here is essential to enable the shoulder complex to move freely.

Scapula

This is a thin flat sheet of bone that provides attachments for the muscles of the shoulder complex and the muscles tethering the scapula to the thoracic cage. On the posterior surface, dividing the superior quarter from the rest, is a ridge of bone, the spine of the scapula, which projects laterally to form the acromion process. A projection, the coracoid process, is at the lateral end of the superior border of the scapula immediately above an expanded oval area, the glenoid cavity.

Humerus

This is a long bone, the shaft cylindrical with each end modified for a specific design of joint. The inferior joint will be described in Chapter 9 - The elbow complex. The superior end of the bone is expanded with a smooth head and two tuberosities, the greater and lesser providing attachments for the rotator cuff muscles. There is a groove between them for the biceps tendon.

Clavicle

The clavicle constitutes the only bony connection between the upper limb and the thoracic cage.

Joints of the shoulder

Glenohumeral

A ball and socket joint between the humerus and scapula. This has a very shallow socket which is deepened by the addition of a triangular labrum attached to the periphery of the glenoid cavity of the scapula.

Sternoclavicular

A large synovial joint divided by an articular disc which is firmly attached below to the cartilage of the first rib and above to the sternal end of the clavicle. It is a saddle joint and this allows, due to the laxity of the capsule and supporting sternoclavicular ligament, movement in all directions including rotation.

Acromioclavicular

A small plane joint between the lateral end of the clavicle and the acromion process of the scapula.

Ligaments of the shoulder

Glenohumeral joint [Figure 8.1]

The capsule of the glenohumeral joint is very lax to allow the joint the maximum range of movement. It is thickened by two ligaments, the coracohumeral and the glenohumeral.

Glenohumeral ligament

This divides into three bands that form a 'Z' shape across the anterior surface. The superior band runs from the upper margin of the glenoid over the humeral head; the middle runs from the upper margin of the glenoid across the front of the humeral head; and the inferior runs from below the humeral head to the anterior glenoid margin. All three bands assist in limiting external rotation of the glenohumeral joint while abduction is limited by the middle and inferior bands.

Coracohumeral ligament

This runs from the coracoid process to the greater tuberosity where the supraspinatus muscle inserts. There are two bands: the anterior assists in limiting extension; the posterior in limiting flexion.

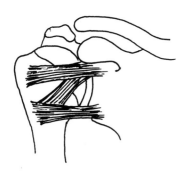

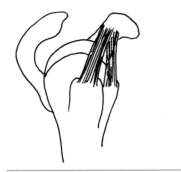

Figure 8.1 The glenohumeral and the coracohumeral ligament.

Sternoclavicular joint [Figure 8.2]

Costoclavicular ligament

This runs from the first rib to the inferior surface of the clavicle. With the subclavius muscle, it assists in restricting elevation of the clavicle.

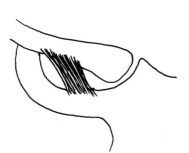

Figure 8.2 The costoclavicular ligament.

Acromioclavicular joint

In addition to the capsule, there are three ligaments that give the joint strength and stability. They are the strong coracoacromial ligament, the acromioclavicular ligament and the medial coracoclavicular ligament.

The coracoclavicular ligament [Figure 8.3]

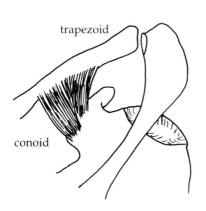

This is divided into two: the conoid and trapezoid ligaments. These very strong ligaments are under a constant state of tension and hold the clavicle down onto the acromion. They run from the coronoid process of the scapula to the inferior surface of the clavicle, are shaped as their names suggest and have different roles.

The conoid ligament restricts anterior movement of the clavicle or retraction of the scapula whilst the trapezoid ligament restricts posterior movement of the clavicle or protraction of the scapula.

Figure 8.3 The coracoclavicular ligament.

The aromioclavicular ligament
This blends with, and supports directly, the joint capsule.

The medial coracoclavicular ligament
This runs from the conoid process medially to the clavicle.

The coracoacromial ligament
Although this is not involved in joint control, it passes from the conoid process to the acromion process and helps form the supraspinatus sulcus.

Bursae around the shoulder

There are a variable number of bursae round the shoulder complex; the more regular and important are identified in Figure 8.4.

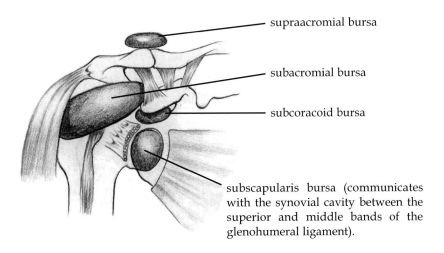

supraacromial bursa

subacromial bursa

subcoracoid bursa

subscapularis bursa (communicates with the synovial cavity between the superior and middle bands of the glenohumeral ligament).

Figure 8.4 Bursae round the shoulder.

There are also bursa behind the coracobrachialis, between the teres major and the long head of triceps, between the anterior and posterior parts of the latissimus dorsi and beneath the infraspinatus.

Muscles of the shoulder

The major muscles of the shoulder complex can be grouped together depending on their action during simple movements. When deciding which muscles are acting in specific functional actions, first decide how the simple movements have been combined, then identify the individual muscles [Tables 1 - 4].

Table 1 The major muscles of the shoulder complex used during flexion and abduction.

Primarily movement at the glenohumeral joint

	Origin	Insertion
0-60° flexion		
Deltoid	Clavicle, acromion, spine of scapula	Deltoid tuberosity of humerus
Supraspinatus	Supraspinatus fossa	Greater tuberosity of humerus [highest facet]
Coracobrachialis	Coracoid process	Medial mid-shaft of humerus
Biceps	Short head: coracoid process Long head: supraglenoid tubercle	Tuberosity of radius
Pectoralis major	Clavicle, sternum, costal cartilages of ribs 2-6	Lateral lip of bicipital groove

Biceps and pectoralis major are very weak flexors of the shoulder

Primarily movement at the scapulothoracic joint [rotation of the scapula]

60-120° flexion		
Trapezius	Superior nuchal line, ligamentum nuchae, S/P C7-T12	Clavicle, acromion, scapular spine
Serratus anterior	Upper 8/9 ribs	Medial margin of scapula

Primarily movement at the glenohumeral joint

0-90° abduction		
Supraspinatus	Supraspinatus fossa	Greater tuberosity of humerus [highest facet]
Deltoid	Clavicle, acromion, spine of scapula	Deltoid tuberosity of humerus
Biceps	Short head: coracoid process Long head: supraglenoid tubercle	Tuberosity of radius

Biceps is a weak abductor of the shoulder

Primarily movement at the scapulothoracic joint [rotation of the scapula]

90-150° abduction		
Trapezius	Superior nuchal line, ligamentum nuchae, S/P C7-T12	Clavicle, acromion, scapular spine
Serratus anterior	Upper 8/9 ribs	Medial margin of scapula

If the arms are flexed above 120° or abducted above 150°, a selection of the following muscles in Table 2 will be involved in the movement. If only one arm is moved, the muscles will produce contralateral spinal side-bending; if both arms are moved then spinal extension, especially in the lumbar spine, occurs.

Table 2 The muscles of the shoulder complex which are involved if the arms are flexed above 120° or abducted above 150°.

	Origin	Insertion
Erector spinae	Iliac crest, sacrum, S/Ps lumbar spine	Ribs, T/Ps of thoracic and cervical spine
Latissimus dorsi	S/P T7-L5, sacrum, iliac crest	Floor of bicipital groove
Serratus posterior inferior	S/P T11-L2	Posterior ribs 9-12
Psoas	T/P L1-4, anterior vertebral bodies, discs	Lesser trochanter of femur
Quadratus lumborum	12th rib T/P L1-4	T/P L1-4, iliac crest
External oblique	Angles of lower 8 ribs	Iliac crest, pubis
Internal oblique	Rectus sheath, costal margin	Lumbar fascia, iliac crest

Table 3 The major muscles of the shoulder complex used during extension.

	Origin	Insertion
Extension		
Latissimus dorsi	S/P T7-L5, sacrum, iliac crest	Floor of bicipital groove
Deltoid [posterior]	Acromion, spine of scapula	Deltoid tuberosity of humerus
Teres major	Lower 1/3 lateral border scapula	Medial lip of bicipital groove
Long head triceps	Infraglenoid tubercle	Olecranon process of ulna
Pectoralis major [sternal head]	Sternum	Lateral lip of bicipital groove

Teres major and long head of triceps are weak extensors of the shoulder and the sternal head of pectoralis major assists when extending the shoulder from flexion.

Hands on: a clinical companion

Table 4 The major muscles of the shoulder complex used during adduction, medial rotation and lateral rotation.

	Origin	Insertion
Adduction		
Pectoralis major	Clavicle, sternum, costal cartilages of ribs 2 -6	Lateral lip of bicipital groove
Latissimus dorsi	S/P T7-L5, sacrum, iliac crest	Floor of bicipital groove
Teres major	Lower 1/3 lateral border of scapula	Medial lip of bicipital groove
Deltoid [posterior fibres]	Acromion, spine of scapula	Deltoid tuberosity of humerus
Coracobrachialis	Coracoid process	Medial side mid-shaft of humerus
Rhomboid major	S/P T2-5	Medial border scapula
Rhomboid minor	S/P C7, T1	Medial border scapula at root of spine
Long head triceps	Infraglenoid tubercle	Olecranon process of ulna

Deltoid [posterior fibres], coracobrachialis, rhomboid major and minor and the long head of triceps are weak adductors of the shoulder.

Medial rotation		
Subscapularis	Subscapular fossa	Lesser tuberosity of humerus
Teres major	Lower 1/3 lateral border of scapula	Medial lip of bicipital groove
Deltoid [anterior fibres]	Clavicle	Deltoid tuberosity of humerus
Pectoralis major	Clavicle, sternum, costal cartilages of ribs 2 -6	Lateral lip of bicipital groove humerus
Latissimus dorsi	S/P T7-L5, sacrum, iliac crest	Floor of bicipital groove
Supraspinatus	Supraspinatus fossa	Greater tuberosity of humerus [highest facet]

Teres major, deltoid [anterior fibres], pectoralis major, latissimus dorsi and supraspinatus are weak medial rotators of the shoulder.

Lateral rotation		
Infraspinatus	Infraspinatus fossa	Greater tuberosity of humerus [middle facet]
Teres minor	Upper 2/3 lateral border scapula	Greater tuberosity of humerus [lowest facet]
Deltoid [posterior fibres]	Acromion, spine of scapula	Deltoid tuberosity of humerus

Deltoid [posterior fibres] is a weak lateral rotator of the shoulder.

Table 5 Muscles of the scapulothoracic joint.

	Origin	Insertion
Elevators		
Trapezius [mid]	Lower ligamentum nuchae, S/P C7-T4	Upper crest of scapular spine
Levator scapulae	T/P C1-4	Superior angle scapula
Rhomboid major	S/P T2-5	Medial border scapula
Rhomboid minor	S/P C7, T1	Medial border scapula at root of spine
Depressors		
Latissimus dorsi	S/P T7-L5, sacrum, iliac crest,	Floor of bicipital groove
Pectoralis major [lower]	Costal cartilages of ribs 4-6	Lateral lip of bicipital groove
Serratus anterior [lower]	Anterior ribs 6-9	Medial border scapula
Pectoralis minor	Ribs 2-5	Coronoid process
Subclavius	Inferior surface clavicle	Superior surface 1st rib
Trapezius [lower]	S/P T4-12	Crest of scapular spine

Serratus anterior, pectoralis minor, subclavius and trapezius are weak depressors of the scapula.

Rotators that move the inferior angle of the scapula towards the thoracic spine		
Levator scapulae	T/P C1-4	Superior angle scapula
Rhomboid major	S/P T2-5	Medial border scapula
Rhomboid minor	S/P C7, T1	Medial border scapula at root of spine
Pectoralis minor	Ribs 2-5	Coronoid process
Pectoralis major	Lower fibres from costal cartilages of ribs 4-6	Lateral lip of bicipital groove
Latissimus dorsi	S/P T7-L5, sacrum, iliac crest	Floor of bicipital groove

Pectoralis major and latissimus dorsi are weak rotators.

Rotators that move the inferior angle of the scapula away from the thoracic spine		
Trapezius [mid]	Lower ligamentum nuchae, S/P C7-T4	Upper crest of scapular spine
Serratus anterior	Anterior ribs 1-8 or 9	Medial border scapula

Protractors of the scapula		
Serratus anterior	Anterior ribs 1-8 or 9	Medial border scapula
Pectoralis minor	Ribs 2-5	Coronoid process
Pectoralis major	Clavicle, sternum, costal cartilages of ribs 2-6	Lateral lip of bicipital groove

Retractors of the scapula		
Trapezius	Superior nuchal line, ligamentum nuchae, S/P C7-T12	Clavicle, acromion and upper crest of scapular spine
Rhomboid major	S/P T2-5	Medial border scapula
Rhomboid minor	S/P C7, T1	Medial border scapula at root of spine
Latissimus dorsi	S/P T7-L5, sacrum, iliac crest	Floor of bicipital groove

Latissimus dorsi is a weak retractor of the scapula.

Differential diagnosis in the shoulder complex

Tables 6 and 7 are not designed to be the means to a definite diagnosis for the commonest musculoskeletal problems in the shoulder complex but identify the commonest and classical symptoms associated with each condition. It is important to remember that every patient is unique; how they react to and interpret their symptoms provides the practitioner with the challenge of making a diagnosis.

Table 6 Muscular conditions and common symptoms.

	Rotator cuff tear	Biceps tenosynovitis	Supraspinatus tear
Age at onset [yrs]	40-50	Any	Any, more elderly
Pain site	Over muscle	Over tendon	Over muscle or tendon
Onset	Sudden when muscle under strain	Sudden	Sudden or insidious
Aggravating factors	No pain unless impingement on lateral rotation and abduction	Use of muscle flexion at elbow or shoulder, supination hand	Abduction of shoulder humeral head impacted under acromion
Relieving factors	Rest, support, protect affected muscle	Pain on flexion and supination	Support, traction, passive abduction
Special tests	Drop arm, empty can	Speed's	Empty can

Table 7 Articular conditions and common symptoms.

	Adhesive capsulitis	A/C joint	Unstable joint
Age at onset [yrs]	Over 45	Any	10-35
Pain site	General over whole shoulder complex	Very localised	General over joint especially anteriorly
Onset	Gradual or sudden	Traumatic or gradual	Traumatic or recurrent problem
Aggravating factors	Any movement towards full range	Pain at end of range on adduction or elevation	Stress on joint, full range of movement
Relieving factors	Support, gentle movement near body	Support of upper limb	Support, rest
Special tests	None	Shear	Load and shift, apprehension

Common pathological conditions of the shoulder

Glenohumeral joint

Infections

Pyogenic
Usually caused by osteomyelitis in the bone local to the joint. This is a less common site than the leg and will affect the upper metaphysis of the humerus. There will be general pyrexia and severe pain. Chronic osteomyelitis is usually a sequel to acute infection with resulting thickened bone structure and a discharge. Possible recurrent episodes of pain.

Tuberculosis
Rare in the UK although becoming more common. Acute pain in the joint with a marked reduction in range of movement.

Arthritis

Rheumatoid arthritis
Occasionally the shoulder is affected, but always with other joint involvement. The joint is stiff and swollen with a slight reduction in range of movement.

Osteoarthritis
Seldom occurs primarily in this joint. It can develop secondary to joint disease, following direct injury, dislocation or surgery.

Ankylosing spondylitis
40% of sufferers have symptoms in the shoulder. There will be gross mobility restrictions in the pelvis, lumbar and thoracic spines.

Mechanical: articular

Recurrent dislocation
The first episode will be between 20-40 years of age, following direct trauma to the shoulder or due to a congenital shallow glenohumeral

socket. The dislocation commonly occurs anteriorly, especially when the shoulder is laterally rotated and abducted.

Adhesive capsulitis
Generally follows either obvious direct trauma or microrepetitive trauma. All ranges of movement will be reduced. The shoulder complex and scapula elevate as a unit on abduction or flexion of the shoulder.

Mechanical: extra-articular

Rotator cuff tear
Complete or partial tear of the muscular cuff, commonly the supraspinatus tendon following trauma. Commonly seen in women over 60 years of age with degeneration of the muscular tendon. Active abduction will cause a painful arc of movement between 60-90°, but the patient will be able to hold their arm above 90° if placed there passively. There is full passive range of movement.

Supraspinatus tendonitis and subacromial bursitis
This can affect any age group but is more common in the elderly. Pain is caused when the supraspinatus tendon or subacromial bursa is pinched or compressed by the humeral head under the acromial process. There will be a painful arc of movement present, eased by traction or gentle passive rotation of the joint.

Supraspinatus calcification
Calcium deposits in the tendon of the supraspinatus particularly in middle-aged adults. Repeated passage of deposit under the acromion process irritates the subacrominal bursa causing pain and tenderness on abduction. A painful arc of movement is present. Passive abduction and traction eases pain.

Biceps tendonitis
Friction on the tendon whilst in its sheath in the groove. There is pain over the anterior shoulder area which is aggravated by use of the muscle, flexion of the shoulder or elbow, or supination of the forearm.

Biceps rupture

Occasionally degeneration and rupture of the tendon occur in middle-aged men. The patient notices a muscle bulge and slight tenderness over the anterior aspect of the shoulder.

Tumours

Benign

Osteoclastoma in the upper humerus, particularly in young adults.

Malignant

The primary lesion is less common than in the leg, appearing in the upper end of the humerus. Usually it is an osteosarcoma in a young adult or child. Secondary deposits from the lung, breast, prostate, kidney, or thyroid. Commonly found especially in the upper end of the humerus.

Acromioclavicular joint

Osteoarthritis

Not common but can occur in patients over 50. Pain and tenderness is localised to the joint line at the limit of acromioclavicular movement.

Subluxation/dislocation

Following direct trauma to the point of the shoulder. There is an obvious step on the acromioclavicular joint line and occasional pain at the limit of shoulder abduction.

Sternoclavicular joint

Arthritis

Occasionally pyogenic, rheumatoid arthritis or tuberculosis.

Subluxation/dislocation

Anterior dislocation following injury. Prominent clavicle with mild pain.

Common extrinsic causes of symptoms

Cervical spine

Prolapsed intervertebral disc, spondylotic changes, cervical rib, upper cord lesion of the brachial plexus, herpes zoster, tumour in the spinal column.

Thoracic spine and ribs

Polymyalgia rheumatica, lower cord lesion of the brachial plexus, pleurisy, angina pectoris.

Abdominal cavity

Referred pain from the diaphragm, liver, spleen, gall bladder or a subphrenic abscess.

Physical examination of the shoulder

Positions and patterns

	Glenohumeral	Acromioclavicular	Sternoclavicular
Resting	55° abduction	arm by side	arm by side
Close packed	full abduction, lateral rotation	90° abduction	full elevation

Active range of movement

	Shoulder	Scapula	Acromioclavicular	Sternoclavicular
flexion	180°			anterior
extension	45-50°	elevation		and
abduction	180°	to		superior 10cm
adduction	30-40°	depression		
rotation			30°	30°
internal rotation	95°	10-12cm		posterior and
external rotation	80°			inferior 3cm

Special tests for the shoulder

Impingement tests

Neer test - Supraspinatus
The patient sits on the treatment table and their arm is forcibly elevated by the practitioner through flexion, jamming the greater tuberosity into the acromion. A positive test will cause pain and indicates overuse to supraspinatus or occasionally biceps.

Reverse impingement test
Used when the patient complains of a painful arc of movement or pain on lateral rotation to test for mechanical impingement under the acromion process. The patient lies supine, the humeral head is pushed inferiorly to disengage, the shoulder is then abducted or laterally rotated. Reduction in pain is a positive test.

Instability tests

Crank apprehension test for anterior dislocation
The patient lies supine and the shoulder is passively abducted to 90° and laterally rotated. A positive test is judged by the patient's look or feeling of apprehension to the movement or resistance to further movement.

Load and shift test
The patient sits with no support. The practitioner stands behind and supports the scapula with one hand while holding the humeral head with the other. The humeral head is seated into the glenoid fossa [the load] then pushed anteriorly or posteriorly [the shift]. Translation of up to 25% of the humeral head diameter is considered normal.

Sulcus test for inferior instability
The patient stands or sits with the arm relaxed to the side. The practitioner distracts the shoulder. An appearance of a sulcus is positive. This can be repeated in slight abduction of between 20-50°.

Scapular stability

The patient sits on the treatment table and the practitioner measures the distance from the inferior and superior angles of the scapula horizontally to the nearest thoracic spinous process. These measurements are repeated in four different positions of the shoulder.

45°   abduction.
90°   abduction with medial rotation.
120° abduction.
150° abduction.

The measurements should not vary by more than 1.5cm from the original measurement.

Winging of scapula

The patient stands facing the wall and presses their outstretched hands onto the wall. On the affected side, the scapula will project posteriorly. This can be caused by a lesion of the long thoracic nerve [serratus anterior weakness: inferior angle rotates clockwise], and the accessory nerve [trapezius weakness: inferior angle rotates anticlockwise].

Acromioclavicular shear test

The patient lies supine with their arm across the anterior chest holding their opposite shoulder. The practitioner palpates the acromioclavicular joint and then exerts a pressure up along the shaft of the humerus towards the shoulder which will shear the joint. Pain or excessive movement indicates a positive test.

Muscle testing

Active resisted movement of the shoulder

When testing and comparing the active resisted movements of the shoulder, it is important to remember that the most powerful movements are adduction and extension. The next strongest are flexion and abduction followed by medial rotation and finally lateral rotation.

Specific muscles can be easily tested as their actions are well documented [see previous tables on muscle action].

Muscle tendon pathology tests

Speed's test [biceps]
The patient sits with their arm to their side and the elbow slightly flexed. The practitioner resists active flexion of the shoulder whilst passively supinating, then pronating, and finally extending the elbow. A positive test causes increased tenderness in the bicipital groove.

Lippman's test [biceps]
The patient sits or stands while the practitioner holds the arm flexed to 90°. The practitioner then palpates the biceps tendon in the bicipital groove 7cm below the glenohumeral joint and moves the tendon from side-to-side. A sharp pain is a positive test.

Empty can [supraspinatus]
The patient stands or sits while the practitioner actively resists abduction beyond 90° without any medial rotation. The shoulder is then medially rotated and angled forward by 30° so the patient's thumbs point to the floor [the empty can position] and abduction is again resisted. Pain in this position is a positive test.

Drop arm [rotator cuff]
The patient sits or stands while the practitioner passively abducts the shoulder to 90°. The patient then slowly returns the arm to their side. Pain or inability to let the arm down slowly indicates a positive test.

Pectoralis major contraction test
The patient lies supine with their fingers interlaced behind their head. The elbows are then allowed to passively drop towards the treatment table. An inability to place the elbows on the treatment table indicates a positive test.

Lift off sign [subscapularis or rhomboid]

The patient stands with their hand on their back trouser pocket with their palm facing posteriorly. An inability to push their hand away from the pocket due to pain is a positive test. If the rhomboids are affected, the medial edge of the scapula may wing slightly.

Chapter 9

The elbow complex

The elbow comprises three closely associated articulations, the humero-ulnar, the humero-radial and the superior radio-ulnar joints. The humero-ulnar is a simple hinge joint that allows flexion and extension while the humero-radial and superior radio-ulnar joints allow rotation that is described as supination and pronation.

The lower end of the humerus is flattened with the articulation for the radius and ulna between two bony processes, the epicondyles. The articular surface of the humerus is divided into the egg-shaped capitulum for the radial articulation and the pulley-shaped trochlea for the ulna articulation. Posteriorly, the olecranon fossa accepts the olecranon process of the ulna while anteriorly, there are two small fossae: the radial for the radial head and the coronoid for the coronoid process of the ulna. Passing posteriorly across the medial epicondyle is a groove for the ulnar nerve.

The superior end of the radius is smaller than the inferior and flattened and disc-like with a narrow neck. There is a large tuberosity for the attachment of the biceps tendon.

The superior end of the ulna is larger than the distal and has two prominent projections: the olecranon and coronoid processes. Together, they bound the trochlea notch that articulates with the humerus. There is a small articular facet for the radial head, the radial notch.

Ligaments of the elbow

There are two main groups of ligaments: the medial and lateral collateral ligaments. Each group originates from its humeral epicondyle origin and fans into three bands: posterior, intermediate and anterior. The medial collateral ligament attaches to the ulna whilst the lateral collateral ligament mainly inserts into the annular ligament that encircles the radial head and is attached to the anterior and posterior borders of the radial notch on the ulna. An oblique cord arises from the tuberosity of the ulna and passes to the radius just lateral to the radial tuberosity.

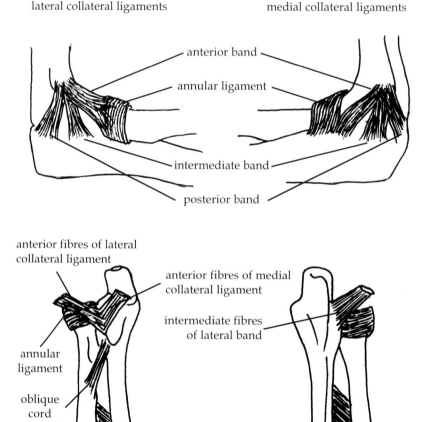

Figure 9.1 The ligaments of the elbow.

Fatty pads around the elbow

There are four fatty pads between the synovial membrane and capsule:-

◆ partly dividing the joint into the humero-radial and the humero-ulnar aspects within a fold of synovial membrane;
◆ over the olecranon fossa;
◆ over the coronoid fossa;
◆ small pads either side of the trochlear notch.

In addition, there are bursae situated between the biceps tendon and radial tuberosity, and between the triceps and the olecranon process.

Muscles of the elbow

The muscles of the elbow complex can be divided simply into flexors and extensors with the muscle belly above the elbow, and supinators and pronators with the muscle belly below the elbow. Biceps and pronator teres have dual roles. The actions of the muscles are shown in Table 1.

In addition, muscles attached to the epicondyles, are primarily associated with the wrist and hand.

Attaching to the medial epicondyle [common flexor origin] and the supracondylar ridge are:-

◆ pronator teres, flexor carpi radialis, palmaris longus, flexor carpi ulnaris.

Attaching to the lateral epicondyle [common extensor origin] are:-

◆ extensor carpi radialis brevis, extensor digitorum, extensor digiti minimi, extensor carpi ulnaris.

Table 1 The muscles of the elbow.

	Origin	Insertion
Flexion		
Biceps	Short head: coracoid process	Tuberosity of radius
	Long head: supraglenoid tubercle	
Brachialis	Anterior humerus	Coronoid process of ulna
Brachioradialis	Lateral supracondylar ridge	Styloid process of radius
	of humerus	
Pronator teres	Common flexor tendon	Mid radial shaft
Extension		
Triceps	Long head: infraglenoid tubercle	Olecranon process of ulna
	Lateral head: posterolateral humerus	
	Medial head: posteromedial humerus	
Anconeus	Lateral epicondyle of humerus	Olecranon process of ulna
Supination		
Supinator	Lateral epicondyle of humerus	Lateral side of radius
Biceps	Short head: coracoid process	
	Long head: supraglenoid tubercle	Tuberosity of radius
Pronation		
Pronator teres	Common flexor origin	Mid radial shaft
Pronator quadratus	Medial side distal ulna	Anterior surface distal radius
Flexor carpi radialis	Common flexor tendon	Base of 2nd, 3rd metacarpals

Common pathological conditions of the elbow

Deformities

Cubitus valgus and cubitus varus

History of previous injury of a fracture with malunion, or interference with epiphysial growth by injury or infection.

Osteochondritis dissecans
The elbow is often affected. Any loose bodies present will cause painful and recurrent locking.

Loose bodies
Synovial chondromatosis will cause painful recurrent locking. Occasionally loose bodies are found in osteoarthrosis or following a fracture.

Infections

Pyogenic
Usually caused by osteomyelitis in bone local to the joint. There is pain and swelling in the joint.

Tuberculosis
A less common site than the knee or other weight-bearing joint.

Arthritis

Rheumatoid arthritis
Commonly one or both elbows will be affected with other joints.

Osteoarthritis
A rare site except after injury or in heavy manual workers. It presents with a slow increase in pain, osteophytic growth and can impinge the ulnar nerve as it passes through the groove in the medial epicondyle.

Haemophilia
Bleeding into the joint is common in a haemophiliac patient, or patient on long-term warfarin therapy with prolonged clotting time.

Neuropathic
A rare form of arthritis eg. Charcot's.

Mechanical: articular

Radial head dislocation
Seen in children between 2-5 years of age following forcible traction to the joint. Often accidental as the parent pulls a reluctant child or prevents the child from falling over.

Mechanical: extra-articular

Olecranon bursitis
Chronic and recurrent pressure on the olecranon process by leaning on elbows or following direct trauma, septic infection or gout. Clinically, bursa is greatly enlarged and the pressure may cause ulnar nerve impingement.

Tennis elbow
A common extensor origin strain particularly in the 35+ age group, following repetitive movements causing local tenderness and pain on gripping, in particular, small objects in the hand. The larger the diameter of the object, the less pain is caused.

Golfer's elbow
A common flexor origin strain particularly in the 35+ age group, following repetitive movements causing local tenderness and pain using the hand.

Ulnar nerve entrapment
Within the groove behind the elbow, resulting in paraesthesia in C8 distribution only in the hand.

Median nerve entrapment
As it passes between the two heads of pronator teres, or as it passes under the ligament of Struthers [found in 1% of population].

Radial nerve entrapment
As it passes between the two heads of supinator. There is weakness in the forearm and hand but triceps is not affected.

Physical examination of the elbow

Positions and patterns

	Humero-ulnar	Humero-radial	Superior radio-ulnar
Resting	70° flexion, 10° supination	full extension, full supination	35° supination, 70° flexion
Close packed	extension with supination	flexion 90°, supination 5°	5° supination

Active range of movement

flexion 145°   extension 5-10°   pronation 85°   supination 90°

The carrying angle is between 5°-15° greater in women to accommodate the wider pelvis. An increased angle is termed cubitus valgus; a reduced angle, cubitus varus.

Special tests for the elbow

Neural entrapment

Ulnar nerve
Tinel's test. Direct pressure on the ulnar nerve in the groove causes neural symptoms in the ulnar distribution in the hand, and local tenderness.

Median nerve
The elbow is passively flexed to 90° and the practitioner actively resists pronation while extending the elbow. A positive test causes neural symptoms in median nerve distribution.

Radial nerve
The elbow is held in slight flexion and the practitioner actively resists supination and extension of the elbow. A positive test causes neural symptoms in the radial nerve distribution.

Muscular tears

Tennis elbow
The patient sits or lies supine and positions their arm at their side, fingers straight, elbow almost in full extension. The patient extends, against resistance, the straight middle finger. Pain over the lateral epicondyle is a positive test. The pain may be reduced by applying pressure just distal to the common tendon origin and repeating the test. In Cozen's test the elbow is stabilised by the practitioner's thumb while the patient makes a fist and attempts to pronate, radial deviate and extend their wrist against resistance. A positive test produces pain.

Golfer's elbow
The patient sits or lies supine while the practitioner palpates the medial epicondyle and passively supinates the forearm and extends the wrist. Pain over the medial epicondyle is a positive test.

Chapter 10

The hand and wrist complex

This is the distal joint complex of the upper extremity, and involves the distal end of the radius, the ulna and the eight carpal bones of the wrist. The distal end of the radius is expanded, with a small styloid process projecting from the lateral border, providing the majority of the articular surface for the proximal row of carpal bones. The distal end of the ulna consists mostly of a rounded small head with a small projection, the styloid process. It articulates with the medial border of the radius, in the ulnar notch, and is separated from the carpal bones by a triangular articular disc. The base is attached to the inferior border of the notch for the distal radio-ulnar joint and the apex is inserted into the ulnar head at the root of the styloid process.

There are two rows of four carpal bones within the wrist: the proximal row comprises the scaphoid, lunate, triquetral and pisiform; the distal row the hamate, capitate, trapezoid and trapezium.

There are two functional joint complexes: the inferior radio-ulnar joint that allows pronation and supination, and the radiocarpal joint where flexion and extension occurs. Within the wrist and part of the radiocarpal complex, there are two distinct rows of joints: between the radius and proximal row of carpal bones, and between the proximal and distal row of carpal bones.

Ligaments of the hand and wrist

Inferior radio-ulnar joint

This joint is supported by the inferior, anterior and posterior radio-ulnar ligaments and articular disc. The anterior and posterior edges of the ligament are slightly thickened and their main functions are to hold the bones in close proximity and restrict supination.

Medial and lateral collateral ligaments

These ligaments pass from the radius [the lateral collateral] or ulna [the medial collateral], and attach to the carpal bones. They restrict ulnar deviation or adduction, and radial deviation or abduction respectively.

Anterior and posterior ligaments

These ligaments fan out from the carpal bones and restrict flexion and extension of the wrist.

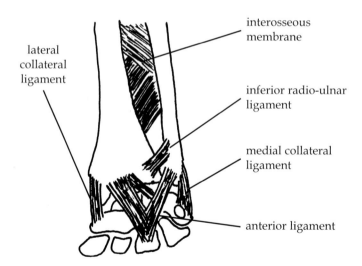

Figure 10.1 Anterior view of the ligaments of the wrist.

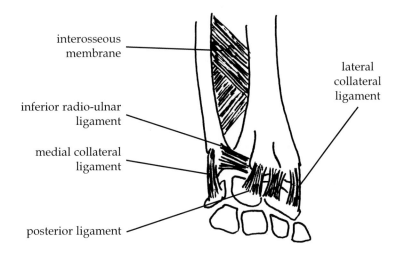

interosseous
membrane

lateral
collateral
ligament

inferior radio-ulnar
ligament

medial collateral
ligament

posterior ligament

Figure 10.2 Posterior view of the ligaments of the wrist.

Interosseous and intercarpal ligaments

Situated between individual carpal bones, they are strong and restrict movement between the carpal bones in each row. There is slightly more movement between the distal and proximal rows of carpal bones than the proximal row and radio-ulnar joint.

Flexor and extensor retinaculum

Although not working to restrict joint movement, these ligamentous structures pass across the palmar and dorsal surfaces to tether the tendons to the wrist during the many and varied movements that the hand performs.

Muscles of the hand and wrist

Tables 1, 2 and 3 outline the major muscles of the area. Figures 10.3, 10.4, 10.5 and 10.6 give an indication of the relative position of tendons from specific muscles as they pass through the wrist.

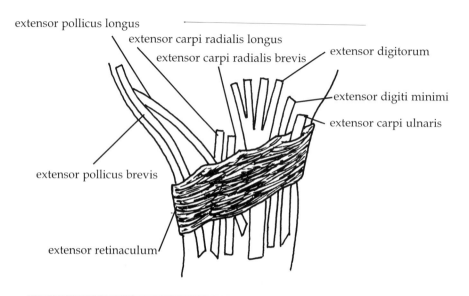

Figure 10.3 The posterior view showing the position of muscle tendons in the wrist.

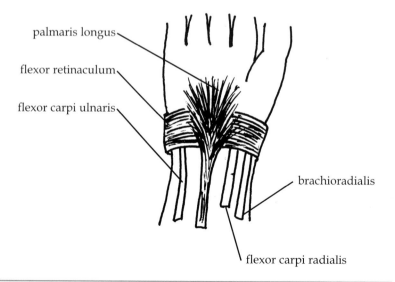

Figure 10.4 The anterior view showing the position of muscle tendons in the wrist.

Table 1 The extension and adduction muscles of the hand and wrist.

	Origin	Insertion
Extension		
Extensor carpi radialis brevis	Common extensor tendon	Base of the 3rd metacarpal
Extensor carpi radialis longus	Lower third of the lateral supracondylar ridge	Base of the 2nd metacarpal
Extensor digitorum	Common extensor tendon	Extensor expansion of digits 2-5
Extensor digiti minimi	Common extensor tendon	Extensor tendon to 5th digit
Extensor carpi ulnaris	Common extensor tendon and ulna	Medial base of 5th metacarpal
Extensor pollicus brevis	Interosseous membrane and distal radius	Base of the proximal phalanx of thumb
Extensor pollicus longus	Interosseous membrane and ulna	Base of the distal phalanx of thumb
Extensor indicis	Interosseous membrane and distal ulna	Tendon for index finger
Adduction [ulnar deviation]		
Extensor digiti minimi	Common extensor tendon	Extensor tendon to 5th digit
Flexor carpi ulnaris	Common flexor tendon, ulnar head	Pisiform, hook of hamate, base of 5th metacarpal
Extensor carpi ulnaris	Common extensor tendon and ulna	Medial base of 5th metacarpal

Table 2 The flexion muscles of the hand and wrist.

	Origin	Insertion
Flexion		
Flexor carpi radialis	Common flexor tendon	Base of 2nd, 3rd metacarpals
Palmaris longus	Common flexor tendon	Palmar aponeurosis
Flexor carpi ulnaris	Common flexor tendon, ulnar head	Pisiform, hook of hamate, base of 5th metacarpal
Flexor digitorum profundus	Upper ulna, interosseous membrane	Base of middle phalanges of digits 2-5
Flexor digitorum superficialis	Common flexor tendon	Distal phalanges of digits 2-5

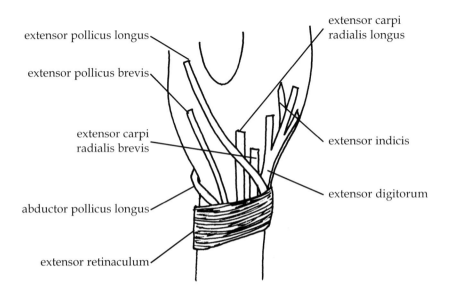

Figure 10.5 Radial aspect showing the position of muscle tendons in the wrist.

Table 3 The abduction muscles of the hand and wrist.

	Origin	Insertion
Abduction **[radial deviation]**		
Extensor carpi radialis brevis	Common extensor tendon	Base of 3rd metacarpal
Extensor carpi radialis longus	Lower third of the lateral supracondylar ridge	Base of 2nd metacarpal
Flexor carpi radialis	Common flexor tendon	Base of 2nd, 3rd metacarpals
Extensor pollicus brevis	Interosseous membrane and distal radius	Base of proximal phalanx of thumb
Extensor pollicus longus	Interosseous membrane and ulna	Base of distal phalanx of thumb
Abductor pollicus longus	Interosseous membrane, radius and ulna	Base of 1st metacarpal
Flexor pollicus longus	Interosseous membrane and radius	Base of distal phalanx of thumb

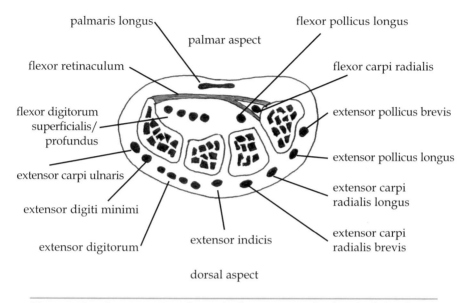

Figure 10.6 Cross-section through the wrist at the level of the flexor retinaculum showing the positions of the tendons.

Common pathological conditions of the hand and wrist

Deformities

Volkmann contraction
A flexion deformity of the wrist and fingers caused by ischaemia of flexor muscles following obstruction of the brachial artery. It is most common in children following fracture or injury to the elbow. The condition develops slowly.

Sudeck's atrophy
Atrophy of carpal bones following simple strain or slight injury [can also affect tarsal bones].

Madelung's deformity
A congenital subluxation/dislocation of the lower end of the ulna. It varies from slight prominence of the lower end of the ulna to complete dislocation.

Kienböck's osteochondritis

This affects the lunate bone. Symptoms include localised pain and reduced strength of grip. In the long-term often leads to osteoarthritic changes in the wrist.

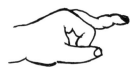

Swan neck deformity

This deformity will only involve the fingers, and is seen in patients with rheumatoid arthritis. There is flexion of the metacarpophalangeal and distal interphalangeal joint with extension of the proximal interphalangeal joint. The result of contracture of the intrinsic muscles of the fingers.

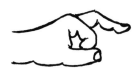

Boutonnière deformity

Due to a rupture of the central tendinous slip of the extensor hood and often seen in rheumatoid arthritis and after direct trauma. The metacarpo-phalangeal and distal interphalangeal joints are extended while the proximal interphalangeal joint is flexed.

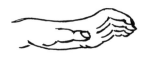

Ape hand

Wasting of the thenar eminence due to median nerve palsy allows the thumb to fall back in line with the fingers. The patient is unable to oppose the thumb.

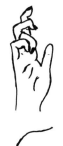

Bishop's hand

Wasting of the hypothenar eminence, interossei and two medial lumbricals due to ulnar nerve palsy. Flexion deformity of the fourth and fifth fingers is the most obvious sign.

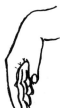

Wrist drop

Wasting of the extensor muscles of the wrist due to radial nerve palsy. The patient is unable to extend the wrist or fingers.

Infections

Pyogenic
In the forearm, infection is usually caused by osteomyelitis in the bone local to the joint. It is rare in this area but there will be pyrexia and severe pain. Chronic osteomyelitis is usually a sequel to acute infection. The bone will be thickened with a discharge and possible recurrent pain. Infection can spread from the infected wound and lead to arthritic changes.

In the hand if superficial infections from cuts and grazes are excluded, infections of the nail-fold [paronychia], pulp-space [Whitlow], thenar space, mid-palmar space or tendon sheath can lead to long-term deformity.

Chronic infective tenosynovitis
This is uncommon in the UK. Histological evidence of tuberculosis.

Tuberculosis
Rare in the wrist but will cause pain, swelling and eventually muscle wasting.

Arthritis

Rheumatoid arthritis
Commonly symmetrical affecting the wrist and joints within the hand. Occurs in women between 20-55 years of age, especially in the metacarpophalangeal joints with ulnar deviation deformity. The joints are red, hot and have reduced range of movement.

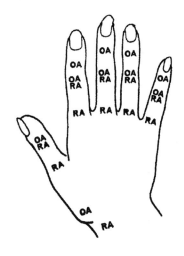

Osteoarthritis
Common in the hand, particularly between 40-60 years of age. The base of the thumb and interphalangeal joints are affected with osteophytes, crepitus and general reduction of movement. Can be in one or both hands but rare in the wrist except after injury.

Figure 10.7 Joints commonly affected by rheumatoid arthritis [RA] and osteoarthritis [OA] in the hand.

Mechanical: extra-articular

Tenosynovitis

This is common in adults between 20-50 years of age, women more than men, whose occupation or hobby demands prolonged periods of repetitive rapid movements of the wrist and fingers. The pain comes on during the activity and remains after completion. There is pain and tenderness over the tendon sheaths.

Soft tissue localised nodular tenosynovitis

A benign tumour arising on the sheath of the tendon or a fibrous extension of the extensor tendon. It can recur unless removed entirely.

De Quervain's tenovaginitis

A nodule in the tendon of abductor pollicis longus and extensor pollicis brevis, especially in middle age. There is a possible history of repetitive strain or pain over the styloid process of the radius.

Trigger finger

A thickening of the flexor tendon at the base of the thumb or a finger. The digit can flex actively but extension from flexion is only achieved passively. A thickening in the tendon can be palpated.

Dupuytren's contracture

A flexion contraction of one or more fingers from thickening of the palmar aponeurosis. It often affects the ring finger first and occurs in men more often than women, between the age of 50-70. Often bilateral and can be hereditary. Associated with excessive alcohol intake.

Rupture of tendon

A history of deep penetrating lacerations, either traumatic or due to self-harm. Occasionally, the tendon is torn from insertion following sudden muscular contraction or stretch.

Median nerve entrapment

Compression in carpal tunnel pain will cause altered sensation in median nerve distribution and muscle weakness, particularly in women between 30-60 years of age. The symptoms are at their worst in the morning and can be eased by holding the arm aloft. Tinel's and Phalen's tests are positive.

Tumours

Benign
Chondromata may interfere in normal growth. Osteoclastoma often affects the lower end of the radius.

Malignant
Rare but will affect the lower end of the radius if anywhere. Generally from the lung.

Others

Ganglion
A cystic swelling on the dorsum of the wrist which can affect adults of any age. It can recur unless excised completely.

Raynaud's disease
Idiopathic paroxysmal bilateral cyanosis of digits, following exposure to cold or a high emotional state. Pain in the digit is associated with changes in colour; the digit will turn white then blue, before finally returning to pink.

Physical examination of the hand and wrist

Positions and patterns

	Resting	Close packed
distal radio-ulnar	10° of supination	5° of supination
radiocarpal	neutral slight ulnar deviation	extension
intercarpal	neutral or slight flexion	extension
midcarpal	neutral slight flexion with ulnar deviation	extension ulnar deviation
carpometacarpal [thumb]	midrange of all ranges	full opposition
carpometacarpal [fingers]	mid flexion and extension	full flexion
metacarpo-phalangeal	slight flexion	
interphalangeal	slight flexion	

Active range of movement

These are a general range and vary between the different joints within the fingers and thumb.

	flexion	extension	abduction	adduction	opposition
wrist	85°	85°	15°	45°	
fingers	80-100°	0-40°	20-30°	0°	
thumb	45-90°	0-5°	60-70°	30°	to little finger

Special tests for the hand and wrist

Carpal tunnel

Tinel's [wrist]
The practitioner holds and passively extends the patient's wrist by placing their thumb over the flexor retinaculum. The practitioner gently taps a patella hammer onto this fixating thumb. A positive test results in sensory disturbance in medial nerve distribution.

Phalen's test
The patient sits and places the dorsum of the hands together in front of their body. The wrists are drawn up, increasing wrist flexion and held for one minute. A positive test results in sensory disturbance in medial nerve distribution.

Chapter 11

The hip

The hip is a ball and socket joint between the femur and the acetabular notch of the pelvic bone. The acetabulum faces laterally and slightly inferiorly. The superior and posterior walls are strong and thick while the inferior is incomplete, forming the acetabular notch. This notch is bridged by the transverse acetabular ligament, a part of the triangular acetabular labrum that deepens the acetabulum and leads into the acetabular fossa, a rough area in the centre of the articular surface.

In the erect position, the femoral head articular surface is not covered completely by the acetabulum and the superior aspect is exposed. For the acetabulum to cover the femoral head articular surface completely, the femur has to be slightly flexed, adducted and medially rotated, the position in which a severely arthritic hip joint is held.

The neck of the femur is angled upwards at 125° to the shaft, and slightly rotated in relation to the condyles. This degree of torsion of the femoral neck is called femoral anteversion and makes an angle of 8-15° in adults between the femoral neck and the femoral condyles when looking down the length of the shaft.

The capsule originates from the acetabular rim in close relation to the insertion of rectus femoris and inserts on the trochanteric line and posterior femoral neck. The capsule is like a cylindrical sleeve with four separate sets of fibres: longitudinal, oblique, arcuate and circular. The ligamentum teres passes from the acetabular notch to the floor of the acetabular fossa, inserting into a small depression on the femoral head, the fovea femoris capitis. In the adult, it is strong but lax and has little mechanical function; in children, it assists with the vascular supply to the femoral head.

Ligaments of the hip

The ligaments of the hip are very strong and can be divided into two groups: anteriorly, the iliofemoral and pubofemoral, and posteriorly, the ischiofemoral.

Anterior

iliofemoral ligament

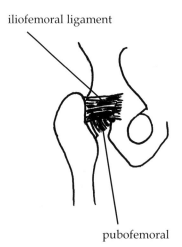

pubofemoral

restricts lateral rotation

Iliofemoral ligament

This is fan-shaped, the apex attached to the anterior superior iliac spine. It has a thickened superior band, the iliotrochanteric ligament, that is 8-10mm thick, and an inferior band. Both attach into the trochanteric line.

Pubofemoral ligament

This originates from the superior ramus of pubis and runs to the trochanteric fossa.

Figure 11.1 The iliofemoral and pubo-femoral ligaments of the hip.

Posterior

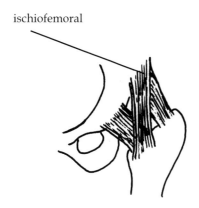

ischiofemoral

Ischiofemoral ligament
On the posterior aspect of the joint, it originates from the posterior acetabular rim and inserts on the inner surface of the greater trochanter.

restricts abduction

Figure 11.2 The ischiofemoral ligament of the hip.

Movements of the hip joint is limited by the tension within these strong ligaments. In the erect position, further extension of the hip is resisted by all the ligaments curling tightly round the femoral neck. Flexion is limited by contact with the abdomen and the general tension in the tissues.

Medial rotation of the hip relaxes all the ligaments except for the ischiofemoral. Lateral rotation is limited by the iliotrochanteric band of the iliofemoral and pubofemoral ligament.

The other leg and the iliotrochanteric band of the iliofemoral ligament limit adduction; the pubofemoral and ischiofemoral ligaments limit abduction.

Muscles of the hip

In Table 1, the major muscles of the area are tabled according to the movement at the hip with some of the muscles that assist the action noted.

Table 1 The muscles of the hip.

	Origin	Insertion
Flexion		
Iliopsoas	T/P L1-4, anterior vertebral bodies, discs, iliac fossa	Lesser trochanter of femur
Tensor fasciae latae	Anterior iliac crest, anterior superior iliac spine	Iliotibial tract
Pectineus	Pecten of pubis	Below lesser trochanter
Adductor brevis	Symphysis pubis, inferior pubic ramus	Upper linea aspera
Sartorius	Anterior superior iliac spine	Medial surface of tibia

Flexion is assisted by adductor longus, gluteus minimus and the anterior part of adductor magnus.

Extension		
Gluteus maximus	Rim of ilium, sacrum, coccyx	Iliotibial tract
Adductor magnus [posterior fibres]	Ischial tuberosity, ischiopubic ramus	Linea aspera

Extension is assisted by semimembranosus, semitendinosus, gluteus medius, the long head of biceps femorus and piriformis.

Adduction		
Adductor brevis	Symphysis pubis, inferior pubic ramus	Upper linea aspera
Adductor longus	Medial superior pubic ramus	Linea aspera
Adductor magnus	Inferior pubic ramus, ischium	Linea aspera
Gracilis	Body inferior ramus of pubis	Medial surface superior tibia

Adduction is assisted by gluteus maximus, the long head of biceps femoris, obturator externus, semitendinosus, iliopsoas and pectineus.

Abduction		
Gluteus medius	Outer aspect of ilium	Greater trochanter
Gluteus minimus	Outer aspect of ilium	Greater trochanter
Tensor fasciae latae	Anterior iliac crest, anterior superior iliac spine	Iliotibial tract

Abduction is assisted by piriformis, sartorius and gluteus maximus when abducted from flexion.

Table 1 continued:-

	Origin	Insertion
Medial rotation		
Gluteus minimus	Outer aspect of ilium	Greater trochanter
Tensor fasciae latae	Anterior iliac crest, anterior superior iliac spine	Iliotibial tract

Medial rotation is assisted by gracilis, posterior fibres adductor magnus, semitendinosus and semimembranosus.

	Origin	Insertion
Lateral rotation		
Gluteus maximus	Rim of ilium, sacrum, coccyx	Iliotibial tract
Iliopsoas	T/P L1-4, anterior vertebral bodies, discs, iliac fossa	Lesser trochanter of femur
Piriformis	Anterior surface of sacrum	Greater trochanter of femur
Quadratus femoris	Ischial tuberosity	Intertrochantic crest
Pectineus	Pecten of pubis	Below lesser trochanter

Lateral rotation is assisted by obturator externus and internus, gluteus medius, sartorius and long head of biceps.

Differential diagnosis in the hip

The hip joint is one joint where a differential diagnosis can be based upon the age of the patient at the time of the onset of symptoms as outlined below [Table 2].

Table 2 Differential diagnoses based upon patient age at onset of symptoms.

Age [years]	Disease
0-2	Congenital dislocation
2-5	Tuberculosis arthritis; transient synovitis
5-10	Perthes' disease; transient synovitis
10-20	Slipped upper femoral epiphysis
20-50+	Osteoarthritis

Common pathological conditions of the hip

Deformities

Congenital dislocation of the hip
One of the commonest congenital deformities, screened for at birth by testing for Ortolani's sign. If missed, a child will present with a short leg and altered gait; the adult with early degeneration of the hip.

Femoral anteversion
Any increase from the normal angle of 8-15° is considered abnormal and will lead to a toeing-in of the foot, medial rotation of the femur or tibia, and lateral patella subluxations.

Femoral retroversion
A reduction of the normal anteversion angle of 8-15° causes a toeing-out of the foot and lateral femoral or tibial rotation.

Coxa valga
An increase in the angle of the neck of the femur from 125° up to 170°. It will cause a long ipsilateral leg with associated posterior pelvic rotation and lateral rotation of the lower limb.

Coxa vara
A reduction in the angle of the neck of the femur from 125° to 100°. It will cause a short ipsilateral leg with associated anterior pelvic rotation and medial rotation of the lower limb. This can be caused by dislocation of the hip.

Osteochondritis [Perthes' disease of the hip]
Unilateral in children from 5-10 years of age. The bony nucleus of the epiphysis undergoes necrosis and loses its trabecular structure. The body weight causes permanent distortion of the femoral head, leading to osteoarthrosis developing early.

Slipped upper femoral epiphysis
Seen in plump boys from 10-20 years of age. In half, both hips are affected. There are selective restrictions into flexion, abduction and medial rotation. The other ranges are normal or increased.

Osteoporosis and fracture of the neck of the femur

Seen in postmenopausal women, more prevalent in the underweight and those who went through the change early. In this group, after a fall it is prudent to assume a fracture even if the original x-ray was negative. Nocturnal pain and severe pain on weight-bearing are indicative of a fracture. A second x-ray to confirm.

Infections

Pyogenic

Uncommon in adults and occasionally seen in children with osteomyelitis. There is generalised illness associated with a severely restricted range of movement of the hip.

Tuberculosis

This condition is becoming more common and frequently affects the hip joint, especially in children between 2-5 years of age and in young adults. There will possibly be a cold abscess in the groin. The patient presents with pain, a limp and swelling.

Arthritis

Rheumatoid arthritis

This is rare in the hip. Other symptoms will be present in other joints: stiffness, swelling, reduced range of movement.

Osteoarthritis

This is common in the elderly or after injury to the joint. In severe cases, the hip is held slightly flexed, medially rotated and adducted.

Ankylosing spondylosis

Gradually develops in the hip following ankylosis of the sacroiliac and lumbar spine. If the hip is affected, this will cause more disability than if the disease affected the spine alone.

Paget's disease

Dull aching pain aggravated by use or immobility, affecting men twice more often than women in the 40+ age group. Of unknown aetiology, it affects, in particular the pelvis, femur, skull, tibia and vertebrae.

Transient synovitis

Found in children under 10 only. The hip range of movement is severely restricted and the diagnosis made only after the attack subsides and other causes have been excluded - in particular, Perthes' disease and tuberculosis.

Common extrinsic causes of symptoms

Disorders of the abdomen and pelvis

Inflammation of the pelvic wall can cause irritation of the obturator nerve, irritation of psoas, iliacus, piriformis or obturator internus. An inguinal hernia or a large abdomen can cause pressure over the femoral nerve in the femoral triangle.

Thrombosis of the lower aorta or branches can give ischaemic pain in the buttock or thigh with pain brought on by activity and relieved by rest. There will be a weak femoral pulse but possibly strong pulses in the foot. The hip has full range of movement with no pain.

Physical examination of the hip

Positions and patterns

Resting	30° flexion, 30° abduction, slight lateral rotation
Close packed	extension, medial rotation, abduction

Active range of movement

flexion	110-120°	**extension**	10-15°	**medial rotation**	30-40°
abduction	30-50°	**adduction**	30°	**lateral rotation**	40-50°

With the hip, much information can be gained from careful observation. Malalignment of the hip can often be seen with the patient standing. Tests can be performed to check the degree of femoral torsion and the angle of the neck of the femur to the shaft.

Femoral anteversion / retroversion

Craig's test

The patient lies prone with the knee flexed to 90°. The practitioner palpates the lateral aspect of the greater trochanter with one hand while medially and laterally rotating the hip until the line of the trochanter is parallel with the table, or reaches its most lateral position. In this position, the angle of anteversion is estimated based upon the angle the lower leg [knee to foot], makes with the vertical. This angle is considered normal when between 8-15°. If greater, a femoral anteversion is present; if less, a femoral retroversion.

Coxa valga / vara

Nelaton's line

The patient is lying supine with the legs straight. The practitioner palpates the ipsilateral anterior superior iliac spine and ischial tuberosity and imagines a line connecting them. The superior aspect of the femoral trochanter is palpated and its position relative to this imaginary line noted. In the normal hip, the superior tip of the greater trochanter should be on the imaginary line. If the superior tip of the greater trochanter is below the imaginary line, a coxa valga is present; if above, a coxa vara is present.

Special tests for the hip

Ortolani's test

Congenital dislocation of the hip in a baby. The baby is placed supine with the hips and knees flexed to 90° with the knees together. The practitioner presses gently backwards while slowly abducting and extending the hips. If the joints are unstable, there is a click as abduction is continued.

Thomas' flexion deformity test

The patient lies supine while the practitioner checks the lumbar lordosis. The practitioner flexes one of the patient's hips and the lordosis reduces. The patient then holds that knee as tight to their chest as possible. Normally the straight leg will remain flat on the table. If a flexion deformity is present in the straight leg, it will lift from the table and if that leg is pushed flat to the table, the lumbar lordosis will increase.

Faber / Patrick's test

The patient lies supine and the knee and hip passively flexed so the foot can rest upon or next to the opposite knee. The practitioner allows the flexed hip to slowly abduct. The knee should reach the table or the tibia should be parallel with the treatment table. In a positive test, the abduction of the hip will be limited by pain which may originate from the hip or iliopsoas spasm.

Trendelenburg's sign

The patient stands and the practitioner palpates the iliac crests. The patient is asked, with the support of a wall if necessary, to lift one foot just off the floor. The practitioner observes the relative positions of the iliac crests. In a negative, normal test, the non-weight-bearing iliac crest should be slightly higher than on the weight-bearing side. In a positive test, the pelvis will drop on the non-weight-bearing side indicating a weak gluteus medius or an unstable hip joint on the weight-bearing side.

Browning's sign [a personal test]

The patient lies supine and the practitioner gently palpates the insertion of the adductor magnus. Tenderness to palpation is an indication that there are osteoarthritic changes within the hip joint.

Muscle tests

Ely's test - tight rectus femoris

The patient lies prone and the practitioner passively flexes the knee. If a tight rectus femoris is present, the hip will flex and lift that side of the pelvis off the table.

Ober's test - tight tensor fasciae latae

The patient lies on the treatment table on their good side with the lower leg flexed at the hip and knee. Standing behind the patient, the practitioner places the upper leg into slight extension and abduction and allows it to gently drop to the table. If contracture is present, the straight leg is unable to reach the table.

Noble's compression test

The patient lies supine and the practitioner flexes one knee to 90°. While the patient slowly straightens the leg, the practitioner places pressure over the insertion of the iliotibial band at the lateral epicondyle. Pain at 30° of flexion of the knee is positive indicating friction between the iliotibial band and the lateral epicondyle of the knee.

Piriformis test

The practitioner stands behind the patient and they lie on their side with the upper hip flexed to 60° and knee flexed, the lower leg straight. The practitioner stabilises the pelvis and applies a downward pressure to the leg. If the piriformis is tight, pain is felt local to the muscle. Resisted lateral rotation of the hip can cause the same pain pattern.

Chapter 12

The knee

The knee is the largest joint in the body, a modified hinge joint with three degrees of movement: flexion, extension and rotation, and an extensive synovium, many bursae and pouches. It is dependent upon ligaments for its stability and as it is situated between two long levers, particularly vulnerable to injuries. The articular surfaces are not congruent; within the space between the bones are two menisci attached to the tibia. In the normal standing position when viewed from the front, the femur makes an angle of approximately 6° from the vertical. The complex comprises two separate joints: the knee or the combination of the tibiofemoral and patellofemoral joints, and the superior tibiofibular joint.

The tibiofemoral joint is between the tibia and the two femoral condyles, the lateral being larger than the medial, united anteriorly by the articular surface for the patella. This surface has a central groove and two facets bordered by prominent lips. The medial facet is deeper whilst the lateral facet is larger and the lip more prominent to prevent dislocation during contraction of the quadriceps muscle.

Of the two menisci, the medial is thicker posteriorly, tethered by the medial collateral ligament and 'C' shaped. The lateral meniscus is more mobile, of equal thickness and 'O' shaped, being separated from the lateral collateral ligament by the popliteus. They are both thicker along the outer margin and thinner on the inner margin. During flexion of the knee, both move posteriorly. The menisci are avascular and poorly innervated and as such have very poor regeneration potential. However, they are vital in aiding lubrication, acting as shock absorbers, making the joint surfaces congruent and reducing friction.

The patellofemoral joint is a modified plane joint with two facets that correspond to the shape of the femur. The patella has the thickest cartilage of any joint in the body and has five facets that come into play depending on the degree of knee flexion. The inferior articulates with the femur from full extension to 20° of flexion, the medial from 20-45° followed by the superior facet from 45-90°. The lateral and odd facet articulates from 90° to full flexion at 135°. The odd facet, situated over the medial epicondyle, is commonly affected by chondromalacia patellae. The plica is a fold of synovial tissue that is situated medially and inferiorly to the patella and is a remnant of tissue pouches found in fetal development. These pouches normally combine to form one large synovial cavity.

The superior tibiofibular joint is a small plane synovial joint that moves in association with movement at the ankle.

Ligaments of the knee

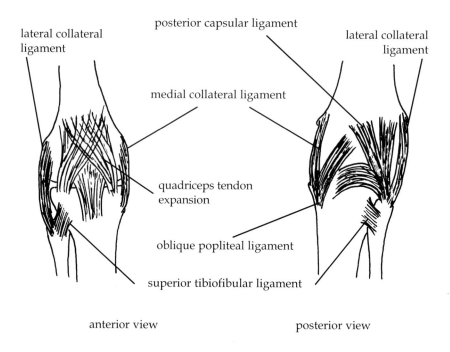

anterior view   posterior view

Figure 12.1 The ligaments of the knee.

The ligaments provide all the strength to the knee joint and are situated between the femoral condyles and the tibia [cruciate ligaments], across the medial and lateral aspect of the joint line [collateral ligaments], and as anterior and posterior thickenings of the capsule. The coronary ligaments assist in tethering the medial and lateral menisci to the tibia. The oblique popliteal ligament is an expansion from the tendon of semimembranosus that reinforces the posterior capsule.

Cruciate ligaments

These are situated deep within the joint. They are extrasynovial and are under tension no matter the degree of flexion or extension of the knee. This tension is increased by medial rotation of the tibia.

The anterior cruciate extends in a superior, posterior and lateral direction twisting on itself as it extends from the tibia to femur. Its main function is to limit anterior shift while the knee is flexed, and to slightly restrict hyperextension of the knee.

The posterior cruciate extends in a superior, anterior and medial direction from the tibia to the femur. It is fan-shaped and is the strongest ligament in the knee. Its main functions are to check hyperextension of the knee and to limit posterior shift of the tibia on the femur.

Collateral ligaments

The medial collateral ligament lies slightly posterior on the medial aspect of the knee and comprises two layers: deep and superficial. The deep layer is a thickened band of the capsule and blends with the meniscus; the superficial layer is strong, broad and triangular, originating near the adductor tubercle and expanding to insert just below the joint line. The lateral collateral ligament is rounded, lying under the biceps femoris tendon running from the lateral epicondyle to the fibular head. It is separated from the lateral meniscus by a small fat pad.

The capsule

This is cylindrical in shape, thickening, particularly posteriorly, with the oblique popliteal ligament and posterior capsular ligament. Anteriorly, the quadriceps tendon expansion over the patella strengthens the capsule.

The strong posterior ligaments working in conjunction with the paired cruciate ligaments limit extension of the knee; flexion is limited by the opposition of the posterior surface of the thigh and tension in the quadriceps expansion.

The powerful but subtle movements of translation, rotation and valgus or varus rotation are resisted by a variety of ligaments.

Anterior translation is resisted by the anterior cruciate ligament with assistance from the collateral ligaments. Posterior translation is resisted by the posterior cruciate ligament with assistance from the collateral ligaments.

Lateral rotation is resisted by the collateral ligaments, while medial rotation is resisted by the cruciate ligaments. Valgus rotation is resisted by the medial collateral ligament assisted by the cruciate ligaments. Varus rotation is resisted by the lateral collateral ligament assisted by the cruciate ligaments.

Ligaments of the superior tibiofibular joint

The ligaments of this simple plane joint are the anterior and posterior tibiofibular ligaments that blend with the capsule of the joint.

Bursae of the knee

There are many bursae situated round the knee joint. They can be classified as communicating with the joint cavity or non-communicating.

Non-communicating bursae are listed below:-

◆ deep infrapatellar bursa	between the patella tendon and tibia;
◆ superficial infrapatellar bursa	between the tendon and the skin;
◆ prepatellar bursa	between the patella and the skin;
◆ anserine bursa	between the medial collateral ligament and adductor tendons.

There are four bursae that communicate directly with the synovial membrane of the knee:-

◆ suprapatellar bursa	between the quadriceps tendon and the anterior femur;
◆ popliteus bursa	between the popliteus tendon and the lateral femoral condyle;
◆ gastrocnemius bursa	between the medial head of the gastrocnemius and medial femoral condyle;
◆ semimembranosus bursa	between the medial femoral condyle and the tendon of semimembranosus.

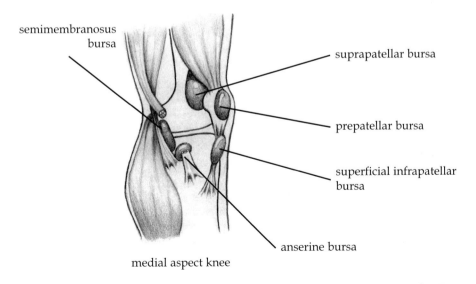

Figure 12.2 The bursae of the knee.

Muscles of the knee

The muscles of the knee can be divided into the powerful flexors and extensors [Table 1], and the rotators [Table 2].

Table 1 The muscles of the knee.

	Origin	Insertion
Flexion		
Semimembranosus	Upper, outer surface of ischial tuberosity	Medial condyle of tibia
Semitendinosus	Ischial tuberosity	Medial tibia (pes anserinus)
Biceps femoris	Long head: ischial tuberosity Short head: linea aspera	Head of fibula, lateral condyle of tibia
Gracilis	Symphysis pubis, inferior pubic ramus	Medial tibia (pes anserinus)
Sartorius	Anterior superior iliac spine	Medial tibia (pes anserinus)
Popliteus	Lateral condyle of femur	Above soleal line of tibia
Gastrocnemius	Medial and lateral heads from above femoral condyle	Calcaneum via achilles tendon

Flexion is assisted by popliteus, gastrocnemius and biceps femoris.

	Origin	Insertion
Extension		
Rectus femoris	Straight head: anterior inferior iliac spine Reflected head: acetabular superior rim	Patella and via patella ligament, tibial tuberosity
Vastus intermedius	Anterior lateral surface of femur	Patella
Vastus lateralis	Lateral lip of linea aspera and gluteal tuberosity	Patella and lateral patellar retinaculum
Vastus medialis	Medial lip of linea aspera	Patella and medial patellar retinaculum
Articularis genu	Anterior femur above patella	Articular capsule of knee
Gastrocnemius	Medial and lateral heads from above femoral condyle	Calcaneum via achilles tendon

Extension is assisted by articularis genu and gastrocnemius.

The rotators are more effective with knee flexion. The popliteus has the primary responsibility of unlocking the extended knee prior to knee flexion.

Table 2 The muscles of the knee.

	Origin	Insertion
Internal rotation		
Sartorius	Anterior superior iliac spine	Medial tibia (pes anserinus)
Gracilis	Symphysis pubis, inferior pubic ramus	Medial tibia (pes anserinus)
Semimembranosus	Upper, outer surface of ischial tuberosity	Medial condyle of tibia
Semitendinosus	Ischial tuberosity	Medial tibia (pes anserinus)
External rotation		
Biceps femoris [long head]	Ischial tuberosity	Head of fibula, lateral condyle of tibia
Tensor fasciae latae	Anterior part of iliac crest, anterior superior iliac spine	Iliotibial tract
Popliteus	Lateral condyle of femur	Above soleal line of tibia

Differential diagnosis in the knee

Direct trauma to the knee

A force into varus or valgus
This will cause injury to the collateral ligament on the opposite side of the joint and possible epiphysial fracture.

A force into hyperextension
This force will cause injury to the anterior and possibly the posterior cruciate ligaments.

A force onto the patella
Direct force on to the flexed knee will cause injury to the posterior cruciate ligament and posterior capsule and direct injury to the patella, patella cartilage or tibial plateau.

Indirect trauma to the knee

Varus or valgus torsion

Indirect force will cause damage to the collateral or cruciate ligaments or cause a meniscoid tear.

Hyperextension

Indirect trauma will cause damage to the anterior cruciate ligament and the posterior capsule.

Common pathological conditions of the knee

Deformities

Osgood Schlatter's disease

This affects boys between 10-14 years of age with pain localised just below the knee over the tibial tubercle and is aggravated by sport and running. The tibial tubercle is enlarged and tender. The condition is limited by fusion of the upper tibial growth plate.

Chondromalacia patellae

Particularly common in young girls with aching or painful knees. The pain is aggravated by going up or down stairs or activities that increase pressure on the articular surface of the patella [especially the odd facet].

Recurrent dislocation of the patella

There is often bilateral congenital absence of the lateral lip of the patellofemoral facet, general ligamentous laxity or genu valgum. It is more common in women or girls. The patella dislocates when on active flexion of the knee, causing muscle spasm that fixes the knee in a degree of flexion. Instant pain relief can be gained by passively extending the affected knee.

Osteochondritis dissecans

Commonly affected, particularly in young men and adolescent boys. There is a recurrent locking with return to full range of movement between attacks.

Loose bodies
Symptoms include recurrent locking with swelling lasting to the next day. 1-3 bodies seen in osteochondritis or chip fractures, 1-10 in osteoarthritis or 50-500 in synovial chondromatosis.

Infections

Osteomyelitis
The bone round the knee is one of the commonest areas affected. There will be pyrexia and severe pain. Chronic osteomyelitis will often follow the acute episode with resulting thickening of the bone structure and discharge with possible episodes of pain.

Tuberculosis
Diffuse knee pain, swelling and wasted quadriceps. An abscess is common.

Syphilitic
Localised swelling, with thickening of the shaft of the tibia. Wasserman's test is positive.

Arthritis

Rheumatoid arthritis
This joint is commonly affected with other joints. The joint will be stiff and swollen, with a slight reduction of the range of movement.

Osteoarthritis
This is the commonest joint in the body to be affected, especially in women who are 'fat, fair and over 40'.

Ankylosing spondylitis
This affects the knee in 15% of cases. It will reduce the range of movement. There are associated symptoms in the pelvis and spine.

Paget's disease

Dull aching pain aggravated by use or immobility, affecting men twice more often than women in the 40+ age group. Of unknown aetiology, it affects, in particular the pelvis, femur, skull, tibia and vertebrae.

Gout

Occasionally affects the knee.

Reiters's syndrome

There is a triad of symptoms often with knee pain, urethritis and conjunctivitis. Especially in promiscuous young males.

Haemophiliac

Bleeding into the knee with recurrent pain is common in haemophiliac patients, or in patients on long-term warfarin medication with increased blood clotting time.

Neuropathic

Charcot's osteoarthropathy, tabes dorsalis.

Mechanical: articular

Medial or lateral meniscus tears

Tears result when the menisci are trapped between the femoral condyle and tibial plateau particularly when the weight-bearing flexed knee is rotated and extended. The onset is initially sudden but can, once a tear is present, become insidious and recurrent. Active movements, in particular full extension, are limited and there is often locking of the knee. The medial meniscus is more likely to tear due to tethering by the medial collateral ligament that restricts its normal movement during flexion of the knee. A positive McMurray's test indicates a torn menicus.

Cyst on the menisci

There is swelling present on the joint line usually on the lateral side which can be seen when the knee is flexed.

Popliteal cyst [Baker's cyst]

A herniation of the synovium posteriorly. The sac extends inferiorly, secondary to persistent effusion of the knee. Associated with osteoarthritis and rheumatoid arthritis.

Mechanical: extra-articular

Rupture of quadriceps tendon
In older men at the patella, or the tibial tuberosity in children. It is caused by unexpected severe contraction of the quadriceps.

Prepatellar bursitis
Recurrent episodes of friction to bursa. Commonly known as housemaid's knee. There is a clearly demarcated swelling.

Plica syndrome
This occurs when the plica is irritated by overuse or injury. Symptoms include pain on full knee flexion, swelling and tenderness over the thickened plica medial to the patella. The knee clicks, locks and there is a history of the knee giving way when forced flexion is applied. Diagnosis usually depends on the exclusion of other conditions that cause similar symptoms. The plica test is positive.

Tumours

Ewing's tumour in childhood or in young adults occasionally causes pathological fractures at the lower end of the femur. Multiple myeloma will occur later in life with the foci in the upper half of the femur. Secondary tumours especially from the lung, breast, prostate, kidney and thyroid develop in the upper half of the femur.

Common extrinsic causes of symptoms

Referred from the hip

Osteoarthritis, slipped upper femoral epiphysis

Ruptured plantaris muscle

A sharp sudden pain in the mid calf during exercise.

Physical examination of the knee

Observation of the knees while standing

Certain malalignments of the knees can be observed while standing. The major ones, together with the associated postures and common areas of compensation, are listed below.

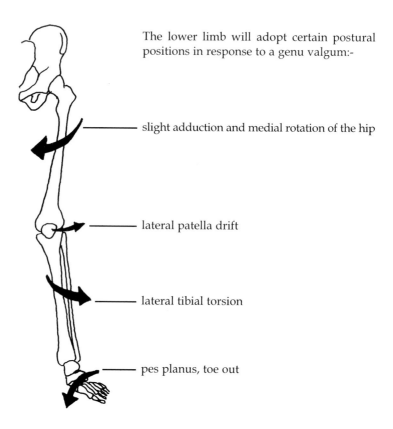

The lower limb will adopt certain postural positions in response to a genu valgum:-

slight adduction and medial rotation of the hip

lateral patella drift

lateral tibial torsion

pes planus, toe out

Figure 12.3 Malalignments of the knee: genu valgum (knock knees).

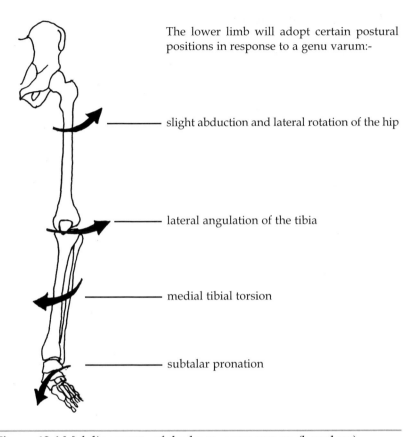

The lower limb will adopt certain postural positions in response to a genu varum:-

——— slight abduction and lateral rotation of the hip

——— lateral angulation of the tibia

——— medial tibial torsion

——— subtalar pronation

Figure 12.4 Malalignments of the knee: genu varum (bow legs).

Positions and patterns

Resting   25° flexion
Close packed   full extension, lateral rotation of tibia

Active range of movement

flexion   0-135° **extension**   0-15°
medial rotation 20-30° **lateral rotation** 30-40°

Special tests for the knee

One plane instability tests

Draw sign

Designed to test the cruciate ligaments. The patient lies supine with the knee flexed to 90° and the hip to 45°. The practitioner perches on the side of the table with the patient's foot placed under their leg for stability. The practitioner holds the tibial plateau, fingers posterior and thumbs anterior, and applies sufficient force to achieve full anterior shift. The range of movement should be no more than 6mm. If excessive, there may be injuries to the anterior cruciate ligament, the posterior capsule or the deep fibres of the medial collateral ligament. If only the cruciate ligament is torn, these other structures will limit the movement. The practitioner pushes the tibial plateau posteriorly to test the posterior cruciate ligament, the posterior oblique ligament or the anterior cruciate ligament.

Slocum test

This combination of tests is conducted in the same position as above except the tibia is first rotated 30° medially, and the tibia drawn anteriorly. If the test is positive, most movement occurs on the lateral side of the knee indicating injury to the anterior cruciate ligament, lateral collateral ligament, posterior cruciate ligament or the iliotibial band. If the test is negative, the knee is rotated laterally 15° and the tibia drawn anteriorly. This time, if the test is positive, more movement occurs on the medial side of the knee indicating injury to the anterior cruciate ligament, medial collateral ligament or the posterior oblique ligament.

Active draw test

As above except the patient attempts to straighten the leg. A positive test occurs when either the anterior or posterior cruciate ligament is torn and the anterior contour of the knee is seen to change. If the posterior cruciate ligament is torn, a posterior sag [tibia drops back on femur under influence of gravity] is evident before the contraction of the quadriceps.

Other tests

McMurray [meniscus]
For this test the patient lies supine with their hip flexed sufficiently to enable the foot to clear the treatment table. The practitioner supports the fully flexed knee and as the test progresses, adds variable degrees of varus and valgus stress to the joint. Pain indicates a positive test.

Lateral meniscus
The knee is fully flexed, and as the knee is passively extended, medial rotation is added. This will test the posterior horn of the meniscus.

Medial meniscus
The knee is fully flexed, and as the knee is passively extended, lateral rotation is added.

Plica test
The patient lies supine with the knee flexed to 30°. The practitioner pushes the patella medially. Pain is a positive test caused by the pinching of the plica between the medial femoral condyle and the patella.

Clark's sign [patellofemoral dysfunction]
The patient lies supine with legs straight. While the practitioner exerts pressure over the patella, the patient gently contracts the quadriceps. Pain is a positive test. Different degrees of flexion of the knee will test different parts of the patella articular surface.

Wilson test [osteochondritis dissecans]
The patient sits with the flexed knee over the edge of the table and actively extends the knee with medial rotation. At about 30° flexion, the pain increases; laterally rotating the knee reduces the pain.

Fairbank's apprehension [patella instability]
The patient lies supine with the knee flexed to 30°. The practitioner gently pushes the patella laterally. An unintentional contraction of the quadriceps in response is a positive test.

Noble compression [iliotibial band friction]

The patient lies supine with their knee flexed to 90° with hip flexion. Pressure is applied to the lateral femoral condyle, while passively extending the knee. Pain occurring at about 30° of flexion is a positive test.

Q angle

This test gives an indication of the angle made between the shaft of the femur and the tibial plateau. The Q angle should be 13° in men, 18° in women. The patient lies supine and their legs are positioned perpendicular to a line drawn connecting the two anterior superior iliac spines. A line is drawn from the anterior superior iliac spine to the centre of the patella, and from the centre of the patella to the tibial tubercle. If increased, it is a sign of genu valgum; if reduced, a sign of genu varum.

Chapter 13

The ankle and foot

This is an intricate area containing 26 bones, 33 joints, 107 ligaments and 19 muscles that combine to hold the structure together whilst allowing it to move in a variety of ways. It is said that feet mirror your general health and consequently this area should be examined with great care as conditions such as arthritis, diabetes and circulatory disorders can exhibit their initial signs or symptoms here. Women have about four times as many foot problems as men, mainly due to fashion and not comfort dictating the design of shoes.

When looked at as a whole, the foot has three arches: the medial longitudinal, the lateral longitudinal and the transverse. The individual shape of bones and joints, the strength of the muscles and support from a network of ligaments generate these arches.

The whole area can be divided into three functional joint complexes:-

Rearfoot	Includes the inferior end of the tibia and fibula, the talus, and the calcaneum.
Midfoot	Includes the articulations between the calcaneum, the talus, navicular and cuboid, and the navicular and cuboid.
Forefoot	Includes the articulations between the cuboid, navicular and the cuneiforms, together with the cuneiform bones, the metatarsals and phalanges.

This chapter concentrates on the structure of the rearfoot and midfoot, but covers all common causes of symptoms in the whole foot.

The rearfoot

The tibiofibular joint
This is not a synovial joint but a syndesmosis or fibrous joint with the concave tibial notch containing fibrocartilage. The fibrous nature of the joint allows movement of the fibula both superiorly and laterally during movement of the ankle.

The talocrural joint [ankle]
The ankle is a modified hinge joint between the distal ends of the tibia and fibula, and the talus. The medial malleolus of the tibia, the lower end of the tibia and the lateral malleolus of the fibula form the articular surface of the ankle. The medial malleolus is slightly smaller and more posterior than the lateral malleolus. The articular surface of the talus is wider anteriorly than posteriorly locking the ankle securely when standing on flat ground.

The subtaloid joint
This lies between the inferior surface of the talus and the superior surface of the calcaneum. It is made up of two separate articular surfaces, allowing the joint to move in three axes of movement.

The midfoot

The midfoot works as a unit. The arches of the foot allow it to adapt to the contour of the ground without placing undue stress on the individual joints. It gives a spring to the step and absorbs the forces of impact from running or walking.

The joints included in this area are the:-

Talocalcaneonavicular joint.	Ball and socket.
Cuneonavicular joint.	Plane.
Cuboideonavicular joint.	Fibrous.
Cuneocuboid joint.	Plane.
Calcaneocuboid joint.	Saddle-shaped.

The forefoot

The most important joints are the intercuneiform joints which are plane joints. The other joints are the hinge joints between the the metatarsals and phalanges.

Ligaments of the ankle and foot

The rearfoot

The inferior tibiofibular joint
The ligaments of this joint are the anterior and posterior inferior tibio-fibular ligaments. These, in association with the interosseous membrane that passes between the tibia and fibula and the fibrous syndemosis, hold the two bones together. While the anterior inferior tibiofibular ligament passes inferiorly and laterally, the posterior tibiofibular ligament passes laterally. They both overlap the joint margin and assist in limiting flexion and extension of the ankle.

The ankle joint
The main ligaments of the ankle are the medial and lateral collateral ligaments, the joint capsule and the inferior tibiofibular ligaments.

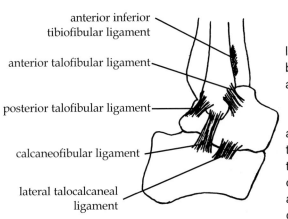

anterior inferior tibiofibular ligament

anterior talofibular ligament

posterior talofibular ligament

calcaneofibular ligament

lateral talocalcaneal ligament

Lateral collateral ligament
This fans from the lateral malleolus in three bands, two to the talus and one to the calcaneum.

The anterior talofibular and the posterior talofibular ligaments pass to the talus while the calcaneofibular ligament attaches to the calcaneum.

Figure 13.1 Lateral view of the ligaments of the rearfoot.

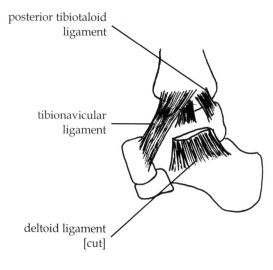

posterior tibiotaloid
ligament

tibionavicular
ligament

deltoid ligament
[cut]

Figure 13.2 Medial view of the ligaments of the rearfoot.

Medial collateral ligament

This fans from the medial malleolus and is divided into two planes, deep and superficial.

The deep plane comprising of the anterior and posterior tibiotaloid ligament attaches to the talus.

The superficial plane, called the deltoid ligament, attaches to the talus, navicular and calcaneum and specifically resists eversion.

The subtalar joint

The two joints that make up the subtalar joint complex are separated by the strong interosseous ligament. This ligament has two bands and passes vertically from the calcaneum to the talus.

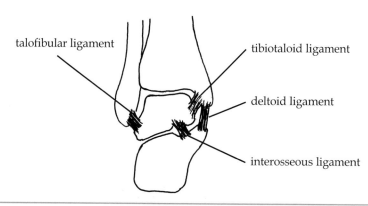

talofibular ligament

tibiotaloid ligament

deltoid ligament

interosseous ligament

Figure 13.3 Anterior section through the talocrural and subtalar joint.

The midfoot

The plantar calcaneonavicular or spring ligament helps in the formation of the talocalcaneonavicular joint and gives attachment to the deltoid ligament of the ankle. The plantar calcaneocuboid ligament helps in maintenance of the longitudinal arch. This ligament originates on the inferior surface of the calcaneum and is divided into deep and superficial layers. The deep layer inserts at the cuboid just proximal to a fibro-osseous tunnel for the tendon of peroneus longus. The superficial layer attaches just distal to this tunnel and sends an expansion to the bases of the last four metatarsals. The other ligaments are short and limit the movement of the joint after which they are named.

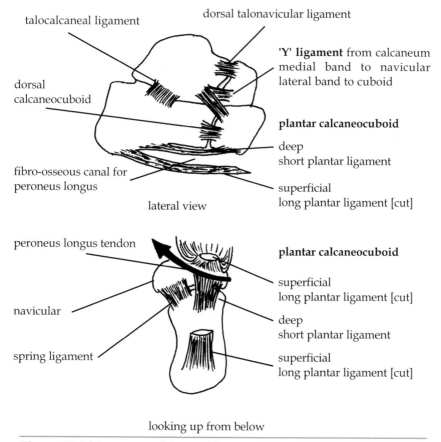

Figure 13.4 Ligaments of the midfoot.

The forefoot

The cuneonavicular intercuneiform and tarsometatarsal joints are all plane joints and their strength depends upon the ligaments, in particular the strong plantar tarsometatarsal and interosseous ligaments, and the shape of the intermediate cuneiform.

Arches of the foot

There are three arches of the foot: longitudinal, transverse and lateral. The longitudinal runs from the calcaneum to the base of the first metatarsal; the transverse from the first metatarsal to the base of the fifth metatarsal; and the lateral from the base of the fifth metatarsal to the calcaneum.

The longitudinal arch is supported by:-

Shape of bones	Navicular [key stone].
Ligaments	In particular the spring and talocalcaneal.
Muscles	Tibialis posterior, tibalis anterior, peroneus longus, flexor digitorum longus, abductor hallucis longus and flexor hallucis longus.

The transverse arch is supported by:-

Shape of bones	Intermediate cuneiform [key stone] and the second metatarsal.
Ligaments	Deep transverse metatarsal ligaments.
Muscles	Abductor digiti minimi, peroneus longus, peroneus brevis, tibialis posterior and adductor hallucis.

The medial arch is supported by:-

Shape of bones	Cuboid [arguably key stone].
Ligaments	Plantar fascia, superficial long plantar ligament.
Muscles	Abductor hallucis, flexor hallucis longus and abductor digiti minimi.

Movement of the foot

Movement of the foot is described as occurring about three axes:-

An axis across the ankle joint.
A vertical axis down the tibia.
A longitudinal axis along the foot.

Movement about the axis of the ankle joint

This is described as dorsiflexion or flexion [toes move upwards towards the shin] or plantar flexion or extension [toes move down away from the shin].

Movement about the vertical axis of the tibia

This is described as adduction [toes in towards the opposite foot] or abduction [toes out away from the opposite foot].

Movement about a longitudinal axis of the foot

This is described as inversion [sole of foot turns in or rotates medially] and eversion [sole of foot turns out or rotates laterally].

Functionally, the foot moves about in a combination of these axes and is described as moving in supination or pronation.

Supination	The combination of adduction, inversion and plantar flexion.
Pronation	The combination of abduction, eversion and dorsi-flexion.

Muscles of the ankle and foot

The muscles of the ankle and foot can be divided according to their action at the ankle [Table 1] and in the foot [Table 2]. During extension of the ankle, tibialis posterior contracts drawing the tibia and fibula together while pulling the fibula inferiorly and slightly into medial rotation. In flexion, the malleoli move apart allowing the talus to move, and the fibula to move superiorly with medial rotation.

Table 1 The muscles of the ankle joint.

	Origin	Insertion
Dorsiflexion		
Tibialis anterior	Lateral tibial condyle, upper lateral surface of tibia	Medial cuneiform 1st metatarsal
Peroneus longus	Upper 2/3 of lateral surface of fibula	Medial cuneiform, base 1st metatarsal
Peroneus brevis	Lower 1/3 lateral surface of fibula	Base 5th metatarsal
Extensor digitorum longus	Lateral tibia, anterior fibula, interosseous membrane	Dorsum of digits 2-5 via extensor expansions
Peroneus tertius	Distal anterior fibula	Dorsum shaft of 5th metatarsal bone
Extensor hallucis longus	Anterior surface fibula, interosseous membrane	Base of distal phalanx of big toe

Dorsiflexion is assisted by peroneus longus and brevis, extensor digitorum longus, peroneus tertius and extensor hallucis longus.

Plantar flexion		
Gastrocnemius	Medial and lateral heads from above femoral condyle	Calcaneum via achilles tendon
Soleus	Head, upper shaft of fibula, soleal line of tibia	Calcaneum via achilles tendon
Plantaris	Lateral femoral condyle	Calcaneum via achilles tendon
Flexor digitorum longus	Mid posterior tibia	Bases of distal phalanges of digits 2-5
Tibialis posterior	Interosseous membrane, posterior fibula, tibia	Navicular medial cuneiform, metatarsals 2-4
Flexor hallucis longus	Lower 2/3 posterior surface of fibula	Base of distal phalanx of big toe

Plantar flexion is assisted by flexor digitorum longus, tibialis posterior and flexor hallucis longus.

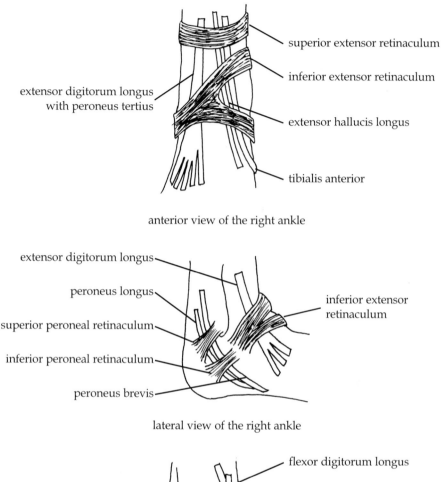

superior extensor retinaculum

inferior extensor retinaculum

extensor digitorum longus
with peroneus tertius

extensor hallucis longus

tibialis anterior

anterior view of the right ankle

extensor digitorum longus

peroneus longus

inferior extensor
retinaculum

superior peroneal retinaculum

inferior peroneal retinaculum

peroneus brevis

lateral view of the right ankle

flexor digitorum longus

tibialis posterior

flexor retinaculum

flexor hallucis longus

medial view of the right ankle

Figure 13.5 Muscles passing over the ankle joint.

Table 2 Muscle action in the foot.

	Origin	Insertion
Supination		
Tibialis anterior	Lateral tibial condyle, upper lateral surface of tibia	Medial cuneiform 1st metatarsal
Extensor hallucis longus	Anterior fibula, interosseous membrane	Base of distal phalanx of big toe
Flexor digitorum longus	Mid posterior tibia	Base of distal phalanges of digits 2-5
Tibialis posterior	Interosseous membrane, posterior fibula, tibia	Navicular medial cuneiform, metatarsals 2-4
Flexor hallucis longus	Lower 2/3 posterior surface of fibula	Base of distal phalanx of big toe

Supination is the combination of adduction, inversion and plantar flexion.

	Origin	Insertion
Pronation		
Peroneus longus	Upper 2/3 lateral surface of fibula	Medial cuneiform base 1st metatarsal
Peroneus brevis	Lower 1/3 lateral surface of fibula	Base 5th metatarsal
Extensor digitorum longus	Lateral tibia, anterior fibula, interosseous membrane	Dorsum of digits 2-5 via extensor expansions
Peroneus tertius	Distal anterior fibula	Dorsum of shaft of 5th metatarsal bone

Pronation is the combination of abduction, eversion and dorsiflexion.

Table 2 groups the muscles by action on the whole of the foot. For ease of understanding the intrinsic muscles of the foot have been omitted.

The following diagram, Figure 13.6, is a cross-section through the lower leg at the level of the ankle joint showing the cut section of the tibia, fibula and talus together with the positions of the tendons.

anterior aspect of the ankle

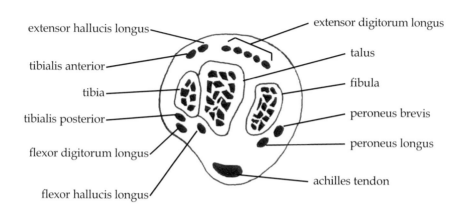

extensor hallucis longus

extensor digitorum longus

tibialis anterior

talus

tibia

fibula

tibialis posterior

peroneus brevis

flexor digitorum longus

peroneus longus

flexor hallucis longus

achilles tendon

posterior aspect of the ankle

Figure 13.6 Cross-section through the talotibial joint of the right leg.

Common pathological conditions of the ankle and foot

Deformities: general

Talipes equinus
Dorsiflexion is limited to under 10° at the ankle joint caused by bone deformity, contracture of gastrocnemius or soleus, talus trauma or inflammatory disease.

Talipes equinovarus [clubfoot]
This is a congenital condition occasionally seen in children with spina bifida or a cleft palate. Treatment is normally undertaken soon after birth and will often leave one foot slightly smaller than the other, altering gait.

Pes cavus
An increase in the height of the longitudinal arch will force the metatarsal heads lower so collapsing the transverse arch. The foot is rigid

with a reduced ability to absorb shock. There are associated claw toes and callus on the plantar surface between the first and fifth metatarsal bones.

Pes planus
The longitudinal arch drops but the flat foot remains mobile. Pain and other symptoms occur while the arch flattens. Once flat, very few symptoms occur in the foot but strain is applied to other joints especially the ankle and knee.

Sudeck's atrophy
Atrophy of tarsal bones following simple strain or slight injury.

Rearfoot deformities

Hindfoot varus
Inversion of the calcaneum with reduced eversion and pronation of the foot can contribute to pes cavus.

Hindfoot valgus
Eversion of the calcaneum with excessive pronation may result from genu valgum. This can give the appearance of pes planus.

Exostosis [heel spur]
At the insertion of the plantar fascia on the calcaneum. This causes localised pain on standing or walking and is treated by a heel pad that removes the pressure on the spur when standing.

Midfoot deformities

Köhler's disease [osteochondritis navicular]
Seen in children 3-5 years of age. There is pain in the midfoot, a slight limp and localised swelling.

Forefoot deformities

Stress fracture
A sudden onset of pain whilst walking/running. There will be localised swelling, with tenderness along the shaft of the bone.

Exostosis
This is due to long-term irritation of bone especially at the base of the big toe, fifth toe or the superior aspect of the navicular.

Hallux valgus
Medial deviation of the first metatarsal. It is more common in women and can be hereditary or caused by ill-fitting shoes.

Polydactyly
An extra digit or toe. There may be other abnormalities present.

Infections

Osteomyelitis
This is due to the frequency of compound fractures to the tibia. It is the commonest site for direct infection leading to osteomyelitis and less common in the fibula. Chronic osteomyelitis is a sequel to the acute episode with thickening of the bone structure and a possible discharge with recurrent episodes of pain.

Tuberculosis
Rare in the foot but will cause a limp, swelling, and wasting of the calf muscles.

Arthritis

Rheumatoid arthritis
The ankles are affected in 70% of cases together with other joints. There is a swollen, tender joint, often accompanied by general ill health.

Osteoarthritis [Hallux rigidis]

This is not associated with hallux valgus but is a degenerative condition of the joint at the base of the first metatarsal. There is a gross restriction of all ranges of movement at the joint, affecting men more than women. It is painful and interferes with the normal gait pattern.

Gout

Affecting men 20 times more than women, and in particular at the big toe. However, it can affect another toe, the ankle, knee or finger. In 90% of cases only one joint is affected with acute irregular pain, swelling and redness.

Reiter's syndrome

Affecting men 20 times more than women. Polyarticular and asymmetrical, and will affect the ankle in 75% of cases. Linked with urethritis, conjunctivitis and plantar fasciitis.

Ulcerative colitis

The arthritis that is associated with this disease will affect the ankle in 50% of cases. There will be abdominal pain and diarrhoea.

Mechanical: extraarticular - general

Post-calcaneal bursitis

Inflammation of the bursa between the tuberosity of the calcaneus and skin. Repeated friction with the shoe leads to chronic pain and swelling.

Calcaneal paratendinitis

Inflammation of tissues covering the achilles tendon from pressure of the shoe, particularly the heel tab present in sports shoes or trainers. There is localised tenderness with full plantar flexion while wearing the shoe over the achilles tendon. It is treated by removing the source of the pressure, the heel tab.

Ruptured achilles tendon

Sudden strain on the tendon when running or jumping. There is sudden sharp pain as if being hit in the calf. The patient is unable to stand on their toes of the affected foot. Thompson's test is positive.

Short achilles tendon
Particularly in women who habitually wear high heels and have difficulty in placing the bare heel to the ground without flexing the knee and taking strain off gastrocnemius.

Mechanical: extraarticular - midfoot and forefoot

Plantar fasciitis
There is pain in the heel under the foot particularly in the middle-aged after prolonged standing. Support of the longitudinal arch eases pain.

Morton's metatarsalgia
A neuroma forms in the digital nerve usually between 3-4 toes. This must be differentially diagnosed from a stress fracture. On standing or walking, pain radiates to the adjoining sides of two toes, aggravated by compression of metatarsal bones. Morton's test is positive.

Tumours

Benign
Chondroma
When associated with dyschondroplasia. The tibia and fibula grow at different rates leading to deformity of the plane of the ankle joint and bowing of the lower leg.

Malignant
Osteosarcoma
Upper metaphysis of the tibia.

Ewing's tumour
The tibia is one of the commonest sites in childhood or early adulthood.

Others

Raynaud's disease
Idiopathic paroxysmal bilateral cyanosis of toes, following exposure to cold or a high emotional state. Pain in the toes is associated with changes in colour: white then blue, before finally returning to pink.

Deep vein thrombosis
The calf is red, hot and very tender. **EXTREME** care is needed when performing Homan's test.

Common extrinsic causes of symptoms

Neural

Diabetic neuropathy, spinal nerve root irritation or compression, spinal stenosis, cord lesions.

Circulation

Intermittent claudication, varicose veins.

Physical examination of the ankle and foot

Positions and patterns

Rearfoot

	tibiofibular	talocrural	subtalar
Resting	plantar flexion	10° plantar flexion	mid range
Close packed	maximum dorsiflexion	maximum dorsiflexion	supination

Midfoot

	midtarsal
Resting	mid range
Close packed	supination

Forefoot

	tarsometatarsal	metatarsophalangeal	interphalangeal
Resting	mid range	mid range 10° extension	slight flexion
Close packed	supination	full extension	full extension

Active range of movement

Plantar flexion	50°	**Dorsiflexion**	20°
Supination	45-60°	**Pronation**	15-30°

Tibial torsion

When looking down the shaft of the tibia, the axis of flexion/extension of the knee and ankle are normally in a slightly different plane. The angular difference is termed tibial torsion, and should be between 13-18° of lateral rotation of the tibia.

To measure the angle, the patient sits on the table with their knees pressed tight against the table edge and feet off the floor. The practitioner palpates the apex of both malleoli visualising a line between. The angle of tibial torsion is the angle that this imaginary line makes with the table edge.

Neutral position of talus

The talus can be placed in the neutral position when the patient is standing, sitting, supine or prone. In the non-weight-bearing positions, the practitioner palpates the head of the talus, anterior and just medial to the malleolli with the thumb and index finger of one hand. The other hand holds the forefoot and after passively placing the foot into slight dorsiflexion, slowly supinates and pronates the foot. With the supination movement, the head of the talus becomes more prominent laterally, with pronation medially. The neutral position of the talus is found when the neck of the talus does not appear to bulge one way more than the other.

In weight-bearing positions the patient stands with the feet slightly apart. The practitioner again palpates the head of the talus anterior and just medial to the malleolli. The patient is asked to slowly rotate their body left and right. While this movement occurs, the head of the talus can be felt bulging medially and laterally. When neither side appears to bulge more than the other, the talus is in the neutral position.

Alignment of the foot

This is the relationship between the leg to the rearfoot, and the rearfoot to forefoot.

Leg to rearfoot

The patient lies prone with their foot over the end of the table. The practitioner marks the leg over the midline of the calf, at the ankle on the midline of the insertion of the achilles tendon and 1cm lower on the midline of the calcaneum. The dots are joined and after the talus is positioned in the neutral position, any angle above the normal 2-8° between the line on the calf and through the calcaneum is noted. If the heel is inverted, a rearfoot varus is present; if everted a rearfoot valgus exists.

Rearfoot to forefoot

The patient lies supine with the feet extending over the end of the table. The practitioner places the talus into the neutral position, then pronates the forefoot to the limit noting the relationship between the vertical axis through the heel and plane through the metatarsal heads. This should be perpendicular: if the medial side is raised, there is a forefoot varus; if the lateral side is raised, there is a forefoot valgus.

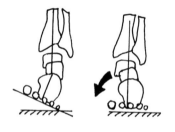

Figure 13.7 Rearfoot varus.

Rearfoot varus [subtalar varus]

This is by far the most common foot disorder and seen in about 85% of the patient population who have rearfoot pronation problems.

There will be a plantar callus under the metatarsals of the second, third and fourth toes, leg fatigue, knee pain and low back pain.

Rearfoot valgus

This is extremely rare but will be associated with severe tibial valgum and excessive subtalar pronation.

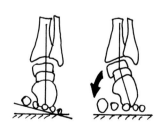

Figure 13.8 Forefoot varus.

Forefoot varus

This is an inverted position of the forefoot relative to the rearfoot at the level of the midtarsal joint. It is due to inadequate frontal plane torsion occurring during normal development of the foot. Calcaneal eversion is required to fully compensate for this deformity.

Forefoot valgus

This is the most common forefoot structural or positional deformity. The forefoot is held in an everted position relative to the rearfoot at the level of the midtarsal joint. Inversion of the lateral border of the foot must occur to allow the forefoot purchase on the supporting surface during the midstance and propulsive phases of gait.

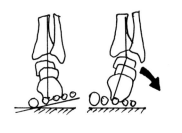

Figure 13.9 Forefoot valgus.

There are two forms of forefoot valgus: flexible and, rarely, rigid. In a flexible forefoot valgus, there is sufficient flexibility in the midtarsal joint to allow the lateral border of the foot to reach the supportive surface during the stance phase of gait. However, in the rigid forefoot valgus, there is insufficient flexibility. To ensure that the lateral border of the foot can reach the ground, rearfoot supination is required.

Special tests for the ankle and foot

Thompson's [rupture of achilles tendon]

The patient kneels on a chair with their feet over the edge of the seat, the practitioner squeezes the calf, and the foot will slightly plantar flex. If there is no movement, it is a positive test.

Swing test [tibiotalar subluxation]

The patient sits on the table with their feet parallel to the ground. The practitioner passively dorsiflexes and plantar flexes the feet in turn and compares resistance to the movement. An increase in resistance in one foot to this passive movement is indicative of a posterior tibiotalar subluxation.

Feiss line [flat feet]

The patient lies supine and the practitioner dorsiflexes the foot and marks the tip of the medial malleolus, the tubercle of the navicular and the base of the big toe, noting the relative position of the navicular to a straight line between the malleolus and big toe. The patient stands and the new position of the navicular tubercle is noted. If it has dropped more than 1cm below the straight line between the big toe and medial malleolus, pes planus is present. Alternatively, the procedure can be performed supine. The foot is passively dorsiflexed, and the imaginary line connecting all three points should be straight. If however, the navicular tubercle is more than 1cm below the line, a pes planus is present.

Homan's test [deep vein thrombosis]

EXTREME care should be taken. The practitioner must first question why it is necessary to perform this test. The patient lies supine and the practitioner passively dorsiflexes the foot. Pain in the calf is a positive sign. If a deep vein thrombosis is present, the calf may be hot, swollen and tender to deep palpation.

Morton's test [neuroma]

The patient lies supine and the practitioner squeezes the forefoot together. Pain is a positive sign.

Chapter 14

Gait assessment

Walking can be described as the art of falling forward - without hitting the ground. Running is the same - only quicker. The gait cycle is defined as a time interval or sequence of movements that occur between two consecutive initial contacts of the same foot. When walking, contact with the ground is maintained; however, when running, there are two phases when contact is lost and the body floats. Normal walking speed will result in approximately 100 steps per minute with the step length averaging 35-40cm. The presence of pain, abnormality or other disability will disrupt the smooth motion of walking, resulting in a limp with a shorter time weight-bearing through the affected side. When walking, the pelvis will rotate, move laterally and vertically up to 5cm, with the maximum vertical movement occuring in midstance. There is a counter-rotation in the thoracic spine that regulates the speed of walking.

Walking

Walking can be divided into the stance phase lasting 60% of the cycle and the swing phase. The stance phase begins with heel strike or initial contact when the forward foot takes the body's weight. At the point of initial contact, the knee is slightly flexed, the ankle plantar flexed and foot supinated. During the midstance phase, the hip moves from flexion to extension, the pelvis rotates anteriorly until the weight is balanced on one leg, then the other leg swings past and the pelvis rotates posteriorly. The hip is in the midrange while the knee extends and the foot moves into slight dorsiflexion. At the terminal phase the other heel strikes and the weight is loaded to that limb; both feet are on the ground. At this point the hip is extended, abducted and laterally rotated, the knee beginning to move from extension to flexion, while the ankle moves from dorsiflexion to plantar flexion. Once the weight is transferred to the other foot, the swing phase begins as the foot is lifted and accelerated forward, past the midswing position when the leg is adjacent to the stance leg to the terminal position when the leg slows in preparation for initial contact and weight transfer. During the swing phase, the hip flexes and moves from lateral rotation to the neutral position while the knee rotates laterally on the tibia in flexion. The ankle is dorsiflexed to allow the foot clearance from the ground.

Running

The mechanics are similar to walking except the two phases, stance and swing, are reduced in length to 40% and 30% of the cycle to accommodate the two float phases each lasting 15% of the cycle. The first float phase occurs at the completion of the terminal stance phase, the leg that was load-bearing accelerating forward and ending when the other leg takes the load. The second float phase begins at the completion of the swing phase, ending with the leg decelerating in preparation for heel strike.

Muscles involved in walking

The process that allows humans to walk upright is very complex, involving all the joints of the body, and not just the joints of the lower limb. Table 1 considers the motion of the different lower limb joints and the action of the main muscle groups during the separate phases of normal walking.

Abnormal gait

There are two primary causes of an abnormal gait: mechanical and neurogenic. The mechanical cause is commonly due to injury, degeneration or changes in leg symmetry, whilst the neurogenic cause can be congenital or acquired.

Mechanical causes

Antalgic
The result of an injury and is designed to protect the damaged tissues or joint. The stance phase on the affected side is shortened, resulting in a

Table 1 The muscles involved in walking.

Phase of gait	Active muscle groups		
	Hip joint	Knee joint	Ankle joint
Stance			
Initial contact	Deceleration of leg by gluteus maximus and hamstrings	Knee flexors	The position of foot is controlled by muscles of ankle
Midstance	Iliopsoas resist extension, gluteus medius stabilises the opposite pelvis	Quadriceps prevent buckling of knee	Plantar flexors control dorsiflexion of ankle
Terminal	Iliopsoas, adductor magnus will stabilise the pelvis and accelerate body mass forward	Gastrocnemius starts knee flexion assisted by quadriceps	Plantar flexors prepare for push off from ground
Swing			
Acceleration	The hip flexors and contralateral gluteus medius begin the leg swing	Hamstrings flex knee, quadriceps resist	Ankle dorsiflexors clear foot from ground
Midswing	Gluteus maximus slows hip flexion	Hamstrings, quadriceps control knee movement	Ankle dorsiflexors keep foot clear from ground
Terminal	Hip extensors decelerate leg	Hamstrings, quadriceps control knee movement	Ankle dorsiflexors place foot on ground

short step length. Often the painful area is supported, if in reach, by the hand. If the pain is from the hip joint, the weight in walking is shifted over the painful joint, reducing the contraction of the abductors hence reducing the pressure on the joint. If the pain is from another lower limb joint, the weight is shifted to the other side.

Arthrogenic

This is caused by the stiffness or deformity of one or more joints. To allow the swing phase to occur, the pelvis will be excessively elevated, the hip circumducted and the ankle excessively dorsiflexed. The step length will be asymmetrical and the painful side will have a shorter and quicker weight-bearing phase.

Leg length discrepancy

There will be a lateral shift of the pelvis to the short side creating a limp. The foot of the short leg will be over-supinated in an effort to lengthen the leg, while the long leg may demonstrate increased flexion at the hip and knee during the swing phase to allow the foot to clear the ground.

Psoatic limp

A variety of hip conditions including Perthes' disease will result in a limp and exaggerated trunk and pelvic movement. The limp may be caused by weakness of psoas and is associated with lateral rotation, flexion and adduction of the hip. The exaggerated movement of the pelvis and trunk assists in moving the thigh through into flexion.

Neurogenic causes

Hemiplegia

The patient will swing the affected limb outwards and ahead in a circle. The affected upper limb will be carried across the body aiding balance.

Parkinsonian

The neck, trunk and knees are flexed. The gait is shuffling with rapid short steps, the arms are held stiffly and the patient progressively moves quicker as if unable to stop.

Ataxic

Poor sensation in the feet so the patient watches their feet and slaps them to the ground. They have poor muscle coordination and balance resulting in a staggering gait with a wide base for stability.

Foot drop

Weak or paralysed dorsiflexors require the foot to be lifted very high by over-flexing the knee or circumducting the hip. The knee is flicked into extension to propel the foot forward and the foot slaps to the ground.

Scissor

Due to spastic paralysis of the hip adductors, the feet are dragged along the ground and forward propulsion is generated by forced rotation of the pelvis or upper body.

Chapter 15

Neurological assessment

The nervous system is usually divided into the autonomic and central nervous systems. The peripheral extension of the central nervous system is further divided into the motor and sensory systems. This chapter is primarily concerned with the interpretation of the general signs and symptoms that arise when the central nervous system is disrupted.

Disruption of neural activity at different levels will produce different patterns of disability, which can present in three simple ways:-

- If the disruption is anywhere on the spinal nerve, there will be a reduction in the normal response. A lower neurone sign.
- If the disruption is from the dorsal root ganglia to the cortex, there will be an increased response. An upper neurone sign.
- If the disruption is within the cortex, there may be a positive phenomena, for example, tremor. An upper neurone sign.

Symptoms that are associated with a neurological problem are varied but include the following:-

- headache, visual disturbance, dizziness;
- radicular linear pain to a limb with or without paraesthesia or numbness;
- specific or general muscle weakness or wasting;
- dysphasia, dysarthria, dysphonia.

A selection of the following signs will accompany an upper neurone problem:-

- ptosis;
- clumsiness;
- confusion;
- altered gait.

There are some signs that only become apparent during the physical examination: rigidity to passive movement of a joint, visual field alteration, nystagmus, muscle wasting or fasciculation.

If any of the symptoms or signs previously mentioned are present, their cause will need to be determined from the case history or special tests during the physical examination. Occasionally, there is not one particular sign but many small indications that the alert practitioner detects which can indicate a neurological problem that needs immediate specialist investigation.

Diseases of peripheral nerves

Multiple sclerosis

The myelin sheath is affected by plaque formation in 0.1% of the population. This will lead to localised inflammation around the nerve axon, initially with widespread symptoms of nerve damage slowly becoming more focused leaving a residual area of permanent dysfunction. A diagnosis requires the demonstration of lesions in more than one anatomical site for which there is no other explanation. The onset of symptoms always occur before 60 years of age and commonly include foot drop, incontinence, optic neuritis, subacute painless spinal cord lesions, subacute loss of function of upper limb or a 6th cranial nerve palsy.

Peripheral neuropathies

Symptoms include bilateral and widespread sensory and motor disturbances, including distal paraesthesia in a glove or sock distribution. There may be distal weakness with reduced or absent reflexes with possible autonomic disturbances. This can occur at any age although it is more common in young to middle-aged adults, especially men.

The following are common and usual causes of peripheral neuropathies:-

Metabolic/endocrine	Diabetes mellitus or chronic renal failure, liver failure.
Toxic	Alcohol.
Inflammatory	Guillain-Barré syndrome, systemic lupus erythematosus, leprosy, polyarteritis nodosa.
Genetic	Charcot-Marie-Tooth, Friedreich's ataxia.
Deficiency states	Vitamin B12, thiamine, folate.
Others	Malignant states, critical illness neuropathy.

Cranial nerves

Bell's palsy
The facial nerve is affected at any age particularly within the facial canal. Symptoms develop over a few hours causing pain around the ear, progressing to loss of movement of that side of the face. There may be some sensory symptoms: a numbness of the skin or a slight loss of taste but the motor symptoms are of more importance to the patient. They cannot smile, close the eye or blow out the cheek on the affected side. Recovery occurs spontaneously within 2-12 weeks. However, in the elderly, the prognosis is poor.

Trigeminal neuralgia
A stabbing acute pain is precipitated by stimulation of the nerve, more often in middle-aged women. The pain lasts up to two minutes and can reoccur several times per day for years.

Diseases of the central nervous system

Viral encephalitis
This can follow a systemic viral infection or vaccination giving rise to malaise, headache, fever, cervical rigidity, and nausea and vomiting.

Meningitis

Common in children and young adults living in close proximity. The symptoms include general signs of systemic infection or flu with a rash that does not blanche on pressure, a stiff rigid neck and photophobia.

Parkinson's disease

A slowly developing disease. The main signs are an involuntary tremor of the hands described as pill rolling, a shuffling gait and lack of facial expression.

Dementia

Mainly beginning between 40-60 years of age. The classical signs include loss of memory, immobility, loss of spontaneity, or restlessness and hyperactivity.

Cerebrovascular vascular accident

Associated with disruption of the vascular supply to the brain by trauma or blockage. Mainly occurs between 50-70 years of age. The symptoms depend on the structures and areas affected.

Physical examination

The practitioner should develop a routine for the sensory and motor systems that can be incorporated into a physical examination. The routine should be logical, symmetrical and fluid:-

Logical	To allow the logical neural pathways to and from the periphery to be followed ensuring no area of supply is missed.
Symmetrical	To enable the patient, in sensory testing, and the practitioner, in motor testing, to compare the normal with abnormal.
Fluid	To enable the patient to relax and thereby reduce the possibility of false positive results that a jerky routine may produce.

Sensory testing

This is divided into testing for disruption within a peripheral nerve, nerve root or central disruption in the brain, brain stem or spinal cord.

Peripheral nerve or nerve root

The sensory loss can be mapped by using light touch and a pin-prick applied as near to the middle of the dermatomes as possible. It is good practice to cover all the dermatomes of the upper and lower limb with light touch as it is gentle and will allow the patient to relax, learn the routine and become aware of the sensation of touch. The routine is then repeated using a sharp object; this noxious stimulus will highlight areas of reduced sensitivity more clearly than light touch. Any areas of reduced or absent sensation are noted and mapped with the sharp object moving in all directions from the area of sensory loss until sensation returns.

By referring to Figures 15.1 and 15.2, an assessment of which nerve root or specific nerve is causing the sensory loss, can be made. If the area of sensory loss or peripheral neural pain is generalised and does not follow a specific nerve or nerve root distribution, it is a central neurological problem or a peripheral nerve neuropathy.

Central disruption within the spinal cord or above

Vibration, using a 128Mhz tuning fork, will test the 'A' fibres in the peripheral nerve and posterior columns of the spinal cord. When performing the test, the practitioner demonstrates what will happen on a normal part of the body, then asks the patient to close their eyes. The practitioner applies a vibrating tuning fork to the malleolus, styloid process or bony prominence of one, then the other limb.

After a variable time period the practitioner carefully stops the vibration. An inability to feel the vibration or its cessation indicates a peripheral neuropathy or spinal cord pathology.

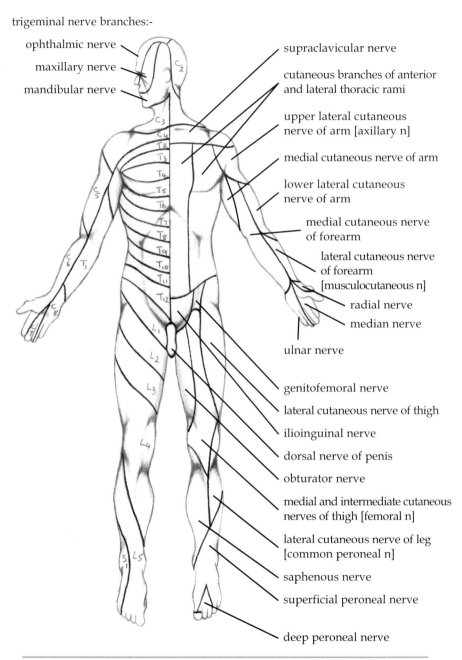

trigeminal nerve branches:-

ophthalmic nerve

maxillary nerve

mandibular nerve

supraclavicular nerve

cutaneous branches of anterior
and lateral thoracic rami

upper lateral cutaneous
nerve of arm [axillary n]

medial cutaneous nerve of arm

lower lateral cutaneous
nerve of arm

medial cutaneous nerve
of forearm

lateral cutaneous nerve
of forearm
[musculocutaneous n]

radial nerve

median nerve

ulnar nerve

genitofemoral nerve

lateral cutaneous nerve of thigh

ilioinguinal nerve

dorsal nerve of penis

obturator nerve

medial and intermediate cutaneous
nerves of thigh [femoral n]

lateral cutaneous nerve of leg
[common peroneal n]

saphenous nerve

superficial peroneal nerve

deep peroneal nerve

Figure 15.1 Anterior view of dermatome map.

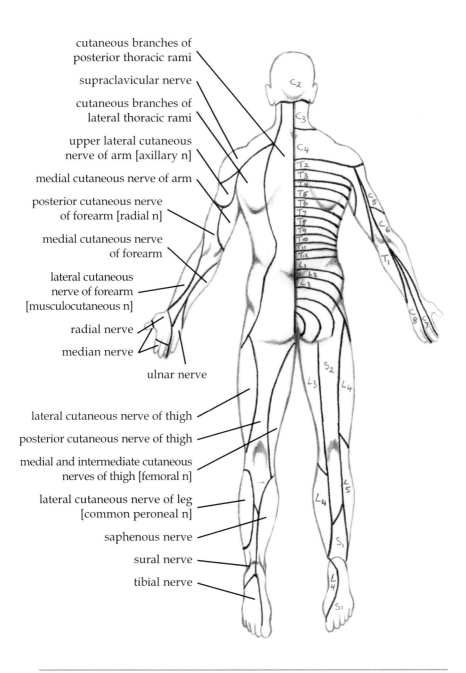

Figure 15.2 Posterior view of dermatome map.

To test the dorsal columns the patient's ability to determine joint position, stereognosis [item identification] or graphaesthesia [number identification] is assessed. If there is a lesion, the patient will be unable to determine the joint position, item or number traced below the level of the lesion:-

Joint position   The patient closes their eyes and the practitioner places individual fingers and toes into varying degrees of flexion [dorsiflexion] and extension [plantar flexion], asking the patient to identify the position.

Stereognosis   The patient is asked to close their eyes and identify an easily recognisable shape placed in their hand.

Graphaesthesia   The patient is asked to close their eyes and the practitioner traces a number or letter onto the patient's hand, ensuring that if the patient had their eyes open they could see a number on their hand the right way round. The patient is asked to identify the number or letter.

Motor testing

This is divided into testing for disruption within a peripheral nerve, nerve root or central disruption in the brain, brain stem or spinal cord. Signs of disruption within the motor system are checked by testing the reflexes and muscle power. The findings will differentiate those from a lower motor neurone lesion or an upper motor neurone lesion.

The commonest signs associated with a lower motor neurone lesion occur on the same side as the lesion and include:-

♦ reduced peripheral reflexes;
♦ weakness in a specific muscle group that is supplied by a spinal nerve root or named peripheral nerve.

The commonest signs associated with an upper motor neurone lesion are more variable, and include:-

♦ uncontrollable jerking of limbs or tremor;
♦ muscle fasciculation or twitching;
♦ generalised weakness of a limb, atrophy or wasting of generalised muscle groups;
♦ impairment of gait, coordination or balance;
♦ involuntary resistance to passive movement of the limb joints and are described as they feel: clasp knife, cog wheel or lead pipe.

The commonest signs associated with a cerebellar lesion are:-

♦ an intentional tremor;
♦ a jerking nystagmus;
♦ ataxic gait.

Reflex testing

Reflexes are an inborn stimulus or response mechanism designed to protect the body from injury. The mechanism is simple and will lead to a glandular response or as described here, a muscular contraction:-

♦ A receptor is stimulated. This initiates an impulse along an afferent neurone to the spinal cord and brain.
♦ A synapse within the spinal segment sends an impulse to an efferent nerve and to the higher centres.
♦ The afferent nerve delivers an impulse to an effector which causes a muscular contraction.
♦ The response is modified by the brain via the vertical corticospinal tract and lateral reticulospinal tract.

Any interruption of this reflex arc within the peripheral nerve will abolish or diminish the response: a lower motor neurone lesion. Any interruption of this reflex arc in the spinal cord or brain will exaggerate the response: an upper motor neurone lesion.

Normal reflexes can be divided into four groups: superficial, deep, visceral and infantile. Pathological reflexes are abnormal and are seen only

Hands on: a clinical companion

with an upper motor neurone lesion. A selection of the commonly tested reflexes and spinal levels involved are described below:-

Superficial membrane

Cornea   A blink following irritation of the cornea cranial nerves V, VII.

Nasal or sneeze   A sneeze following irritation of the nasal membrane cranial nerves V, VII, IX, X.

Pharyngeal   Gagging following irritation of the pharynx cranial nerves IX, X.

Superficial dermal

Abdominal   Subcutaneous muscle tenses when an area of the skin is lightly stroked - spinal nerves T7-12.

Cremasteric   Elevation of the testicle upon stroking the inner thigh - genitofemoral L1.

Plantar   Plantar flexion of the toes when the plantar aspect of the foot is stroked - tibial S1/2.

A diminished or absent superficial reflex when associated with exaggerated deep reflexes and positive pathological reflexes will indicate an upper motor neurone lesion.

Deep muscular

Suddenly stretching the muscle under test by striking just proximal to the point of insertion with the patella hammer gives a reflex contraction of the muscle. The site the patella hammer should strike is described below with the nerve and spinal levels involved:-

Maxillary   Tip of the relaxed lower mandible - cranial nerve V.

Biceps   Near insertion at the anterior aspect of the elbow - musculocutaneous C5/6.

Triceps   Near insertion at the posterior aspect of the elbow - radial C6/7/8.

Periosteoradial   On insertion of the brachioradialis at the lateral aspect of the wrist - radial C5/6.

| Patella | Inferior to the patella on the patella tendon - femoral L2/3/4. |
| Achilles | Posterior aspect of the ankle on the achilles tendon or on the ball of the foot, with the foot held in dorsiflexion - tibial S1/2. |

A reduced or absent reflex may result from peripheral nerve disease or entrapment. An exaggerated reflex shows a lack of inhibition by the higher centres and may indicate an upper motor neurone lesion.

Visceral [or organic]

These are protective reflexes that occur normally. Their absence indicates an upper motor neurone lesion:-

Pupillary	Bright light shone in one eye causes constriction of the pupil - cranial nerve II. [When the other pupil reacts it is called a consensual light reflex and is dependent upon central connections.]
Oculocardiac	Pressure over the eye ball causes slowing of the heart rate - cranial nerve V, X.
Bladder/rectal	Increase in pressure results in a normal urge to urinate or defecate - pudendal S2/3/4.

Infantile

These are found in the normal infant, for example, sucking and swallowing, grasp, rooting, tonic neck. They disappear as the infant develops and grows. They may be absent in cerebral birth injury. In cases of cerebral palsy or in mental retardation, they may remain longer than usual.

Pathological or abnormal reflexes

These are only seen when there is an upper motor neurone lesion present allowing certain primitive reflexes that are usually suppressed by cerebral inhibition return.

Lower limb

Babinski reflex   On stroking the sole of the foot, the toes move into dorsiflexion [normal in babies under 6 months].

Upper limb

Gordon's finger sign   Pressure over the pisiform bone causes extension of flexed fingers or thumb and index finger.

Hoffmann's sign   Clawing movement of the hand when the practitioner flicks the relaxed distal phalanx of the index finger.

Head

McCarthy's sign   Percussion on the supraorbital ridge causes constant blinking. The normal patient will blink several times before stopping.

Muscle testing

To determine if there is a neurological cause for the muscle weakness, the following two screening routines can be used. The first is a general but rapid screening routine; the second tests individual muscles. Table 1 lists the possible causes of the subjective findings in the motor screening examination.

Table 1 The possible causes of muscular symptoms.

Findings	Neurological cause
Increased reflexes	Upper motor neurone lesion or motor neurone disease
Reduced reflexes	Lower motor neurone lesion
Specific muscle tone reduced	Lower motor neurone lesion
General muscle tone increased	Upper motor neurone lesion
Proximal generalised muscular weakness	Myositis
Distal weakness, pathological reflexes	Spinal cord compression
Distal generalised muscular weakness	Peripheral neuropathy
Fasciculation of muscle fibres	Anterior horn cell disease, possible motor neurone disease
Mixed findings that do not fit expected pattern	General neuropathy

The patient lies supine on the examination table and is asked to perform the specific movements listed below against the resistance created by the practitioner. The practitioner makes a subjective assessment as to the strength exhibited by the patient. If weakness on one side is present, a nerve root problem at that level is indicated.

- C1   FLEXION NECK
- C2   EXTENSION NECK
- C3   SIDE-BENDING NECK
- C4   SHRUGGING SHOULDERS
- C5   ABDUCTION OF SHOULDER
- C6   FLEXION ELBOW/ EXTENSION WRIST
- C7   EXTENSION ELBOW/ FLEXION WRIST
- C8   FLEXION FINGERS
- T1   ABDUCTION/ADDUCTION FINGERS

- L2   FLEXION HIP
- L3/4   EXTENSION KNEE
- L4   DORSIFLEXION AND INVERSION ANKLE/FOOT
- L5   EXTENSION HALLUX
- S1   PLANTAR FLEXION AND EVERSION OF ANKLE/FOOT
- S1/2   PLANTAR FLEXION

To determine where a specific spinal nerve is damaged, the strength of individual muscles it supplies can be compared with the opposite and surrounding muscles. Any muscle whose neural supply is distal to the site of damage will become weak and the site of damage can be estimated, as the order of supply of muscles by named nerves is known.

Table 2 lists the major muscles in order of their innervation by the named peripheral nerves with the nerve root identified.

Table 2 The major muscles in order of their innervation by the named peripheral nerves with the nerve root identified.

Upper limb		Lower limb	
Circumflex nerve		**Femoral nerve**	
Deltoid	C5/6	Sartorius	L2/3
Musculocutaneous nerve		Quadriceps	L2/3/4
Biceps	C5/6	**Obturator nerve**	
Coracobrachialis	C5/6/7	Adductors	L2/3/4
Brachialis	C5/6	**Sciatic nerve:**	
Radial nerve		**[Tibial division]**	
Triceps	C6/7/8	Hamstrings	L4/5, S1/2
Brachioradialis	C5/6	Gastrocnemius	L5, S1/2
Extensor carpi	C6/7	Soleus	L5/S1
radialis longus		Tibialis posterior	L4/5, S1/2
Extensor carpi	C6/7/8	Flexor digitorum longus	L4/5, S1/2
radialis brevis		Flexor hallucis longus	L4/5, S1/2/3
Extensor digitorum	C6/7/8	**[Peroneal divison]**	
Extensor carpi ulnaris	C6/7/8	Peroneus longus	L5/S1
Extensor pollicis longus	C6/7/8	Peroneus brevis	L5/S1
Extensor indicis	C6/7/8	Tibialis anterior	L4/5
Supinator	C6/7/8	Extensor digitorum longus	L4/5, S1/2
Abductor pollicis longus	C6/7/8	Extensor hallucis longus	L4/5, S1/2
Extensor pollicis brevis	C6/7/8		
Median nerve			
Pronator teres	C6/7		
Flexor carpi radialis	C6/7		
Palmaris longus	C7/8/T1		
Flexor digitorum	C7/8/T1		
superficialis			
Flexor pollicis longus	C7/8/T1		
Ulnar nerve			
Flexor carpi ulnaris	C8/T1		
Flexor digitorum	C8/T1		
profundus			

Chapter 16

Muscle pain

Problems with muscle can be separated into conditions affecting the nerve supply [covered in the previous chapter], the neuromuscular junction, muscle tissue and others. Most of these are the direct result of a musculoskeletal injury or rheumatological disease process but may be due to vague non-specific conditions such as fibromyalgia, myalgic encephalomyelitis [M.E], restless leg syndrome or vague cramps. Rarely, they may be the presenting features of serious underlying systemic diseases, carcinomatosis or vasculitis.

Neuromuscular junction

Myasthenia gravis
This has an insidious onset with very mild symptoms, fatigability being characteristic preventing repeated or maintained contraction of striated muscle. Patients are between 15-50 years of age [women more than men] and it runs a relapsing remitting course especially in the early years. The first symptoms often include intermittent ptosis and diplopia but it can also affect chewing, swallowing and speaking.

Disease of muscle

Muscular dystrophy
Several inherited disorders [Table 1] are characterised by progressive degeneration of groups of muscles without the involvement of the nervous system. Wasting and weakness is generally symmetrical, with no fasciculation or sensory loss. Muscular reflexes are not lost until the late stage.

Table 1 Types of dystrophy.

Type of dystrophy	How inherited	Age of onset	Affected muscles
Duchenne	X-linked recessive	3-10 yrs	Proximal legs arms, then general
Limb girdle	Autosomal recessive	10-30 yrs	Pelvic or shoulder girdle or both
Facioscapulohumeral	Autosomal dominant	10-40 yrs	Facial, shoulder girdle, serratus anterior
Dystrophia myotonica	Autosomal dominant	any age	Temporalis, facial, sternomastoid, distal limbs, myotonia

Metabolic myopathy

Acute and generalised muscle weakness usually presents in childhood or young adults. It may develop in association with metabolic disorders, particularly glucose, lipid or mitochondrial. Fasting may increase symptoms. However, they are usually reversible.

Endocrine myopathy

Endocrine conditions such as hyperthyroidism, hypothyroidism, Cushing's syndrome or Addison's disease can cause generalised muscular weakness, which is more proximal and especially in the pelvic girdle. Motor neuropathy may be seen in diabetes. Treatment of the underlying condition eases the muscular symptoms.

Toxic myopathy

Alcohol or medication [including steroids, diuretics] can cause a wide range of muscular symptoms from generalised weakness to necrosis. Removal of the offending chemicals results in rapid improvement of the symptoms.

Myositis

An inflammatory muscle disease that occurs either in isolation or associated with a typical rash over extensor surfaces of joints and eyelids. Weakness typically affecting the proximal muscle groups ensure that actions of getting up from a chair, climbing stairs or reaching above shoulder level are difficult.

Fibromyalgia

Also know as fibromyositis, fibrositis or myofascial pain syndrome. It is a benign condition that is diagnosed only by the elimination of the other possible causes of the patient's symptoms, there being no specific tests to confirm the diagnosis. It is possible that it is an extreme variant of M.E. The following must be present before a diagnosis can be made:-

- ◆ widespread pain of at least three months' duration at 11 of 18 defined tender points that are not trigger points [Figure 16.1];
- ◆ a deep aching, radiating, gnawing, shooting or burning pain that increases with activity, cold, damp weather, anxiety and stress;
- ◆ morning stiffness with pain, improving during the day but increasing during the evening;
- ◆ fatigue but no associated muscle weakness.

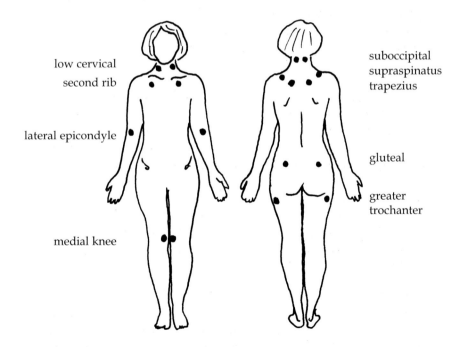

Figure 16.1 The tender areas in fibromyalgia.

Presenting symptoms include:-

Musculoskeletal	Multiple painful areas, facial muscle pain or aching, fatigue, reduced exercise tolerance.
Cerebral	Impaired memory and concentration, irritability, sleep disturbances, non-restorative sleep, dizziness and headaches.
Dermal	Itching and rashes, brittle nails.
Gastrointestinal	Bloating, constipation/diarrhoea, irritable bowel syndrome.
Genitourinary	Increased menstrual and uterine cramps, bladder infections, chronic cystitis.
Miscellaneous	Eye irritations, tinnitus, vertigo, increased sensitivity to light/sound/smell.

Myalgic encephalomyelitis [ME] or chronic fatigue syndrome
This is a chronic disorder which leaves the patient suffering from intense lethargy, mental confusion and muscle and joint pain. It can only be diagnosed by the elimination of other causes for the symptoms, and when the following diagnostic criteria are present:-

- fatigue after minimal effort not eased by rest or sleep;
- fluctuation of symptoms from day-to-day, a tendency for relapses and remissions over months;
- malaise and cognitive dysfunction are invariably present.

The presenting symptoms include:-

Cerebral	Depression, sleeping disorders, irritability, mental confusion, anxiety, headache.
Musculoskeletal	Severe fatigue after minimal effort lasts for days or months, not eased by rest. Muscle aching generally in the lower back or lower limbs.
Miscellaneous	Glandular swelling and sore throat.

Differential diagnosis for fibromyalgia and M.E.

The following conditions must be ruled out before a diagnosis of fibromyalgia or M.E. can be made.

Osteoarthritis
Can coexist with fibromyalgia and M.E. There may be confusion, particularly in the elderly.

Rheumatoid arthritis
Presents with tender joints not tender muscle points.

Hypothyroidism
Can cause widespread muscle aches, depression and fatigue.

Systemic lupus erythematosus
Most patients have a rash and a raised ESR.

Multiple sclerosis
Plaque formation affects function of muscles or sight.

Sjögren's syndrome
An autoimmune condition characterized by dry eyes and mouth.

Lyme disease
Only in later stages will it be confused with fibromyalgia.

Drugs and alcohol
Fatigue can be a side-effect of many medications or abuse of alcohol/illicit drugs. Caffeine withdrawal can produce depression, fatigue and headache.

Polymyalgia rheumatica
Pain, prolonged morning stiffness in the girdle areas. Responds to corticosteroids.

Infectious mononucleosis
Patients complain of joint pain, sore throat, swollen glands and fatigue.

Myasthenia gravis
Progressive inability to sustain a maintained or repeated muscle contraction.

Irritable bowel syndrome
Abdominal bloating which increases in the day. Symptoms are eased by defecation.

Depression disorders
Links between psychological disorders and these conditions are very strong.

Chapter 17

Joint pain

There are three primary causes of joint pain or arthritis:-

♦ the normal ageing or degeneration of the articular cartilage surface with the associated thickening of subchondral bone and formation of osteophytes. This process begins by the early 40s and slowly becomes more pronounced towards old age. The level of pain experienced, frequently bears little relationship to the level of degeneration of the articular surface;

♦ an inflammatory response to an excessive external force or to prolonged repetitive microforces;

♦ an inflammatory response to a systemic pathological disease process. This type of arthritis generally begins for no apparent reason, has a prolonged course with intermittent remissions and associated systemic symptoms. Upon resolution the risk of osteoarthritis developing is increased in the affected joints.

The following descriptions for joint pain have been used: one joint affected is monoarticular, while more than one joint is polyarticular [the term pauciarticular can be used to describe the involvement of between two and five joints and polyarticular for six or more joints]. The following simple flow diagram [Figure 17.1] can assist in identifying possible causes of the joint pain.

When considering a patient presenting with joint pain, the following features need to be explored during the case history process:-

1. Number of joints affected.
2. Pattern of joint involvement.
3. The patient's age at the onset of the pain.
4. Associated systemic symptoms.

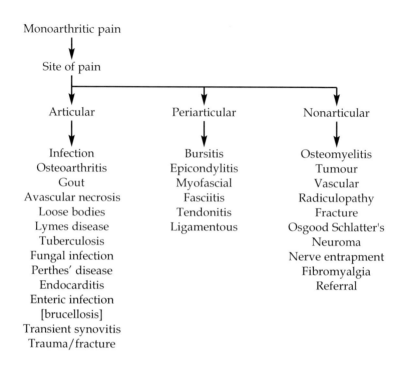

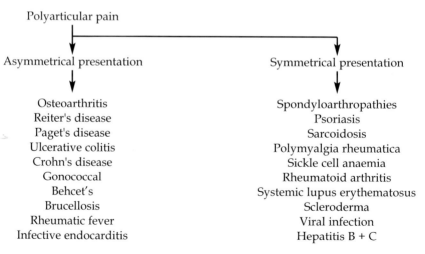

Figure 17.1 Flow chart depicting possible causes of joint pain.

1. Number of joints affected

Monoarticular pain

With a patient presenting with pain in one joint, it is important initially to determine from which tissues the symptoms are originating: within the joint [articular]; associated with the joint [periarticular] or no association with the joint [nonarticular].

Nonarticular

There are numerous conditions that can cause symptoms over a joint, both local and distal. Local conditions include osteomyelitis, tumours [both soft tissue and bony], fractures, specific nerve entrapment, localised visceral pain and referral from an adjacent joint. Distal conditions will generally produce nonspecific symptoms and include radiculopathy, cardiovascular insufficiency, referred neural pain from the spine, viscera or distal joint.

Periarticular

These are tissues that are specifically associated with the joint but are outside the synovial cavity. They include the joint capsule and ligaments, local fascia, bursae, tendons and associated muscles.

Articular

There are five probable causes of a patient presenting with a painful, hot, tender and swollen joint:-

- degeneration of the joint;
- localised direct trauma;
- infection;
- crystal arthritis;
- reactive arthritis.

Degeneration

Although this may be expected in patients over 50, other possible causes of the pain should always be ruled out. In the younger patient, the degeneration may be the result of trauma, repetitive microtrauma, or following an active rheumatological process.

Trauma

This can be an obvious single acute event, a chronic repetitive injury or microtrauma to the joint.

Infection

This must be ruled out before any other cause of the pain is considered. The presence of fever, rigors, or bone infection near the joint will indicate that infection is the probable cause of the pain. The infective agent can reach the joint directly following a penetrating wound, via the vascular system or spread from local osteomyelitis.

Crystal arthritis [gout]

This affects men 20 times more than women between the ages of 30-60 years. The pain is generally recurrent with the initial onset of symptoms occurring for no apparent reason. There is a tendency for recurrent attacks with variable periods of remission. An attack can be triggered by diet, alteration in the production or excretion of uric acid, or the trauma of physical exercise.

Reactive

Following an enteric infection in young adults or inflammatory bowel disease. The generalised systemic disease process associated with brucellosis can give rise to joint pain.

Brucellosis follows contact with infected cows, goats or sheep, or the drinking of raw untreated milk or cream. It can affect a person at any age especially between 20-40 years of age and arthritis occurs in 30% of cases. It affects the knee, hip or shoulder, often affecting the back and sacroiliac joints. Arthritis follows several months of general ill health.

Polyarticular pain

This is defined as pain in two or more joints either with an asymmetrical or a symmetrical pattern of distribution throughout the body. The causes of the pain can include a wide range of systemic, inflammatory, metabolic and degenerative conditions. It is important to remember that conditions that are classically polyarthritic or symmetrical in nature can present early in the disease process with monoarthritic pain or asymmetrical joint involvement.

2. Pattern of joint involvement

Asymmetrical presentation

Osteoarthritis
This may be expected in the elderly, primarily on the dominant side affecting particularly the hip or knee. Other possible causes of the pain should be ruled out.

Paget's disease
There is a dull aching pain aggravated by use or immobility, affecting men twice more often than women in the 40+ age group. An unknown aetiology will affect in particular the pelvis, femur, skull, tibia and vertebrae.

Reiter's disease
This presents as a triad of symptoms: arthritis, urethritis and conjunctivitis, especially in sexually promiscuous males. The usual onset is between 20-40 years of age, affecting primarily the knee, ankle and feet.

Enteropathic
The onset of arthritis is between 25-55 years of age and affects the knee, ankle or other peripheral joints. This type of arthritis is associated with ulcerative colitis or Crohn's disease. Arthritic episodes last one or two months and generally resolve after three attacks. In ulcerative colitis, the arthritis is more common with widespread involvement of the gut and appears in the first few years. In Crohn's disease the arthritis is more

common when the small bowel is involved. Associated symptoms include diarrhoea, rectal bleeding, abdominal pain and weight loss.

Behcet's disease
A syndrome of unknown origin, characterised by a triad of oral ulceration, genital ulceration and iritis. Erythema nodosum frequently occurs. Arthritis occurs in 60% of cases especially in the knee or ankle and can be symmetrical or asymmetrical.

Symmetrical presentation in adults

Viral
This type of arthritis is seen in patients with hepatitis before jaundice appears, particularly young adults abusing drugs or following a blood transfusion.

Rheumatoid arthritis
Commonest between the age of 20-55 years but can present from 16 or up to 70 years. 6% of women are affected. Initially it affects small joints of the hands and feet. Occasionally, it can be monoarticular, restricted to the knee or other large joint.

Ankylosing spondylitis
A chronic condition of the sacroiliac joints and spine leading to progressive calcification of the spinal ligaments, affecting men five times more than women. The onset is between 15-30 years of age and can affect the hips or peripheral joints. It can be associated with iritis and aortic incompetence.

Polymyalgia rheumatica
Affects the 60+ age group, women three times more than men, in the shoulder girdle and pelvis. The primary symptom is severe morning stiffness that lasts at least one hour. Corticosteroids result in rapid symptomatic relief. The condition resolves after 2-4 years but occasionally, medication is required for life.

Psoriatic arthritis

The skin disease is associated with arthritis in 10% of cases. The severity of psoriasis is no indicator of the likely onset of arthritis. The arthritis commonly affects the small joints of the hands in patients between 20-30 years of age mimicking rheumatoid arthritis. The skin lesions will precede the arthritis by many years.

Systemic lupus erythematosus

A multi-system disease with polyarticular pain similar to rheumatoid arthritis. Associated with a butterfly rash on the face, vasculitic lesions on the fingers or mucous membrane lesions in the mouth. Often fever, non-specific gastrointestinal symptoms, cardiovascular, neurological, renal or respiratory symptoms are present.

Sarcoidosis

A condition characterised by granulomatous inflammation of the lymph nodes, spleen, liver and lungs. The arthritis occurs in 10% of cases between 20-30 years of age, affecting the knees and ankles and can last for years with relapses and remissions. It will eventually subside. Other systemic symptoms include Raynaud's phenomenon, oedema, telangiectasis, skin pigmentation, ulcers on the fingers and legs and dysphagia.

Scleroderma

A condition characterised by inflammation of the subcutaneous connective tissue, affecting the 20-50 age group, women three times as often as men. Commonly affects fingers, resembling rheumatoid arthritis in the beginning, although the arthritis abates within the first year of the condition.

Symmetrical presentation in children

Juvenile idiopathic arthritis

Defined as an arthritis that begins before the 16th birthday.

Still's disease

This disease becomes chronic with remissions and relapses. However, the prognosis is generally good especially in cases when the onset is acute. Associated with fever and rash.

Juvenile rheumatoid arthritis
This is similar to the adult disease, with involvement of small joints in the hands and feet. It particularly affects girls between 12-16 years of age.

Ankylosing spondylitis
This particularly affects the lower limb, the knees, ankles and feet of boys from 9-12 years of age.

Sickle cell anaemia
The initial symptoms generally appear before the 10th birthday. In particular, it affects the Afro-Caribbean race, especially of tropical Africa. Joints of the hands or feet are commonly affected, although the condition migrates to other joints. Although the joint pain subsides spontaneously, the patient's life span is considerably reduced by the disease process and punctuated by chronic anaemia, intermittent jaundice, leg ulcers and abdominal pain.

3. Age at onset of arthritic pain

The age of onset of symptoms is another useful tool that can assist when differentiating between the various pathological and non-pathological causes of arthritic pain [Table 1].

Osteochondritis
Occasionally called osteochondritis juvenilis which is a term used to describe specific conditions of the developing bony nuclei in children. The bony centre becomes temporarily softened, deformed by the normal weight through that bone. Then after a variable time it rehardens in the deformed shape. Table 2 lists the common sites, names, ages and duration of the active disease processes.

Table 1 Age at onset of symptoms as a useful tool to differentiate between the causes of arthritic pain.

Age	Conditions									
0-20	Osteochondritis									
10-20		A/S	R/A							
20-30		A/S	R/A	SLE	Sarcoidosis	Psoriatic	Reiter's	Enteric		
30-40			R/A	SLE	Sarcoidosis	Psoriatic	Reiter's	Enteric	Gout	
40-50		Paget's	R/A		Sarcoidosis	Psoriatic		Enteric	Gout	O/A
50-60			R/A					Enteric	Gout	O/A
60+	Polymyalgia rheumatica		R/A							O/A

A/S	Ankylosing spondylitis	R/A	Rheumatoid arthritis
O/A	Osteoarthritis	SLE	Systemic lupus erythematosus

Table 2 The common sites, names, ages and duration of osteochondritis.

Site	Name	Age	Duration
Centre of a single vertebral body	Calvé	2-10	2-3 months
Navicular bone	Köhler	3-5	2 yrs
Upper epiphysis femur	Perthes'	5-10	2 yrs
Ring epiphyses of several vertebral bodies	Scheuermann	13-16	2 yrs
Head of 2nd or 3rd metatarsal bone	Freiberg	14-18	2 yrs
Lunate bone	Kienböck	Adult	2 yrs

4. Associated systemic symptoms

In Tables 3, 4 and 5 the systemic symptoms that are associated with the more common rheumatological conditions are listed. In addition, the other important factors such as incidence, joints affected, signs and symptoms are tabulated for easy comparison.

Table 3 The systemic symptoms associated with the more common rheumatological conditions [symmetrical presentations].

	Rheumatoid arthritis	Ankylosing spondylitis	Systematic lupus erythematosus	Sarcoidosis
Incidence	6% females, F3:1 Onset 16-70 Common 20-55	0.4% males, M5:1 15-30yrs Family history 6%	F9:1 20-40 yrs USA Negroes	F3:1, peak 20-30 10% with arthritis
Joints	75% hands/feet 30% large joints, ultimately knee, ankle, shoulder and cervical spine	Sacroiliac to spine, shoulder and hip in almost half, occasionally peripheral joints	Like rheumatoid arthritis	Knee, ankle, often elbow, wrist, shoulder, hand, occasionally feet, hip, spine
Symptoms	Insidious onset, joint pain and prolonged morning stiffness, general ill health, fatigue	Gradual onset of low back aching with/out pain, morning stiffness	Sudden onset, pain and stiffness, aggravated by sun, stress, 50% have morning stiffness	Sudden or gradual pain and swelling, morning stiffness
Signs	Swollen tender joints, muscle wasting round joints	Reduced all range of movement, reduced chest expansion, tender bony points	50% have no signs; slight swelling or tenderness, most have fever, weight loss	Red, warm, swollen joints, reduced range of movement, occasionally fever
Course	Occasionally episodic, persistent, eventually burns out leaving osteoarthritic changes	Stiffness increases over years, reduced mobility in hips may disable	70% survive 5yrs 50% 10yrs	Chronic for years with relapses/ remissions, slight deformity
Associated symptoms	Tenosynovitis and carpal tunnel, soft tissue nodes, synovial cysts, Baker's cyst ligamentous laxity especially odontoid peg	Iritis	Butterfly rash on face, Osler's nodes, splinter haemorrhages, mucous lesions, vasculitic lesions on fingers	Peripheral lymphadeno- pathy, cutaneous sarcoid iritis

Table 4 The systemic symptoms associated with the more common rheumatological conditions [monoarthritic gout and more symmetrical presentations].

	Gout	Polymyalgia rheumatica	Psoriatic arthropathy
Incidence	M20:1, 30-60 yrs, 50% regular alcohol drinkers	F3:1, 60+ yrs, rare 40+	M=F, 20-50 yrs, 10% with psoriasis develop pain
Joints	Mainly big toe, occasionally ankle, knee, other toes, fingers, single joint	Shoulder girdle, often pelvis/lumbar spine, hips and knees	Mainly hand 10% get ankylosing spondylitiis
Symptoms	Prodromal irritability, sudden onset of pain at 3-6am History of surgery, trauma, drugs, exercise	Acute onset pain, severe morning stiffness, malaise and weight loss	Acute or chronic onset, no morning stiffness
Signs	Red, hot, swollen, very tender joint, local oedema, fever in attack	Reduced movements in affected area, may improve in the day	Acute red, hot, swollen joint, occasionally iritis, atlantioaxial subluxation
Course	Unrelenting for days, reoccurs irregular times, arthritis becomes chronic with deformities	Spontaneous resolution after 2-4 yrs, responds in days to corticosteroids	Recurrent, progressive, mild unless deformities occur
Associated symptoms	Obesity 50%, hypertension, 50% renal stones	Temporal arteritis	Nail changes, hyperkeratosis, occasionally hyper-uricaemia

Table 5 The systemic symptoms associated with the more common rheumatological conditions [asymmetrical presentations].

	Osteoarthrosis	Paget's disease	Reiter's disease	Ulcerative colitis Crohn's disease
Incidence	F2:1, 20% population affected, peak 50 yrs	M2:1, 40+ yrs, often family history	M20:1, 20-40 yrs	M=F, peak 25-55 yrs 25% of patients develop arthritis
Joints	Commonest knee and hip, also hand, low back, ankle Most severe on dominant side	Hip, knee, lumbar spine, thoracic spine	Knee, ankle and feet Also affects shoulder, wrist, elbow, hip, spine	Knee and ankle, often wrist, elbow, fingers, 1-3 joints attacked, may migrate
Symptoms	General morning stiffness, then pain increases during pm or after inactivity	Dull ache, aggravated by use or immobility, stiff after rest	Acute onset pain, swelling, dysuria and penile discharge, occasionally pain in heel	Sudden onset pain, swelling often associated with relapse of underlying disease
Signs	Bony swelling, tender, crepitus, pain at limit of mobility	Joints warm with reduced movements, crepitus in hip, knee; bony swelling	Red, hot, tender joint in acute stage, pyrexia	Pain limits all movement; effusion, abdominal pain, diarrhoea
Course	Chronic, progressive, variable	Chronic, progressive, in end similar to osteoarthritis	First attack resolves after 6 mths, some develop spondylitis	1-2 months between attacks, complete resolution after 1-3 attacks
Associated symptoms		Large skull, deafness, bowed tibia, kyphosis	Urethritis, conjunctivitis, achilles tenosynovitis or plantar fasciitis	Abdominal pain, rectal bleeding, diarrhoea, weight loss, fever, occasionally erythema nodosum and buccal ulceration

Chapter 18

Head pain

Head pain or headache is a very common presenting symptom in the clinical environment. It can be associated with many different conditions from local neural, dental, auditory or musculoskeletal problems to generalised cardiovascular, respiratory, gastrointestinal or renal problems. Due to the association with potential pathological conditions, great care must be taken when taking a case history, especially when questioning the patient about their current and past medical history. As in the following chapters on abdominal and chest pain, it is prudent to assume a serious cause for the headache and concentrate on ruling this out during the case history process. Once an initial diagnosis has been reached, a decision must be made as to whether this condition constitutes a red flag to further evaluation. As mentioned in Chapter 1, the red flag may be total, requiring immediate referral to hospital or a general practitioner, or partial, allowing the examination process to continue with a referral if necessary to the patient's general practitioner in the near future.

Based upon the assumption that a headache affects a specific area of the head and has identifying features that vary with the cause, there are six factors that need to be established before an initial diagnosis can be made. These six factors each give vital information about the headache and hence its cause:-

1. The site of pain.
2. The patient's subjective description of the pain and its cause.
3. The speed of the headache's onset and past headache history.
4. The time of day of the maximum pain.
5. The effects of posture on the pain and other aggravating or relieving factors.
6. Any associated symptoms or signs of systemic disease.

1. Site of pain

The site of pain can generally be described as occurring over a specific cranial bone [Table 1].

Table 1 The site of head pain with common causes and red flag areas.

Area	Common causes	Red flag causes
Frontal	Eye strain, suboccipital muscle tension, sinus infection	Giant cell arteritis
Parietal	Constipation, hysteria	Meningitis, intracranial tumour, giant cell arteritis
Temporal	Migraine, temporomandibular joint	Auriculotemporal neuralgia, ear infection
Occipital	Cervical spondylosis, eye strain	Hypertension, occipital neuralgia
Facial	Sinus infection, dental caries	Trigeminal neuralgia, tonsil or adenoid infection, tumour, tongue

2. Patient's subjective description of the pain and its cause

The commonest descriptive terms used by patients are listed in Table 2.

Table 2 A patient's description of the headache pain and its cause.

Description	Cause
Throbbing/pulsating	Generally vascular in origin, migraine, arterial hypertension, intracranial malformations
Tight constricting band/pressure	Emotion, stress or tension induced
Constant dull/steady ache or pain	Head injury, intracranial mass or haematoma, bone tumour or abscess

3. Speed of the headache's onset and past headache history

Headaches, like any other pain, can occur recurrently or as a single episode. When the headache is recurrent, questions should be directed as to the frequency of the attacks and if specific triggers are known [Table 3].

Table 3 The frequency of headaches related to their common causes.

Frequency	Common causes
Single episode, acute pain	Head trauma, impending cardiovascular accident, subarachnoid haemorrhage, acute infection [sinus, meningitis, middle ear], giant cell arteritis
Recurrent, monthly	Hormonal, migraine, stress/tension, constipation
Recurrent, weekly	Migraine, constipation, stress/tension
Recurrent, daily	Cluster, trigeminal neuralgia, glossopharyngeal neuralgia, eye strain, hypertension

4. Time of day of the maximum pain

The causative factor of the headache will determine when in the day the symptoms begin. As a general rule of thumb, the earlier the pain starts, the more serious the cause [Table 4].

Table 4 The time of day of headaches related to their common causes.

Time of day for onset	Common causes
Night	Intracranial disease, cluster headache, osteomyelitis, nephritis, migraine
Early morning	Hypertension, migraine, sinus infection, excessive alcohol, cluster headache, sleeping position
Afternoon or evening	Eye strain, suboccipital muscle tension, rebound headache, excessive caffeine

5. Effects of posture on the pain and other aggravating or relieving factors

Bending over tends to increase the pain of a headache caused by swelling of pain-sensitive tissues - for example, a sinus infection or hypertension. Lying flat can aggravate a migraine headache.

6. Associated symptoms or signs of systemic disease

With most headaches, there are frequently associated symptoms which relate specifically to either the underlying cause or the specific type of headache [Table 5].

Table 5 Associated symptoms related to the underlying cause or specific type of headache.

Type of headache	Signs	Symptoms
Migraine		Nausea, photophobia, pallor, fluid retention
Cluster	Ipsilateral sweating	Nasal congestion or discharge
Hypertension	Elderly, cervical spondylosis, vertebral artery insufficiency	Cough aggravates
Psychogenic	Anxiety, depression, loss of appetite	Severe bilateral constant pain eased by massage of neck, disturbed sleep pattern
Ear	Discharge, deafness	Tinnitus
Dental	Dentures, gingivitis	Difficulty eating or chewing
Temporomandibular joint	Clicking, inability to open mouth fully	Pain on eating, moving jaw; locking of jaw

Figure 18.1 gives an indication to the different causes of headache in the area of the different bones of the skull.

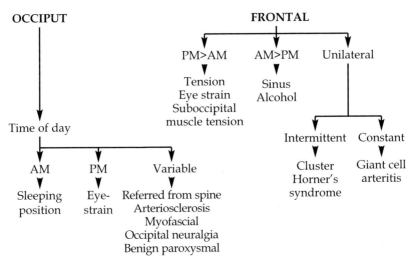

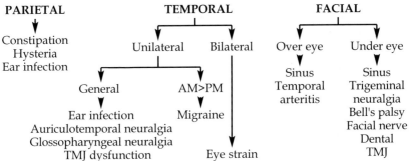

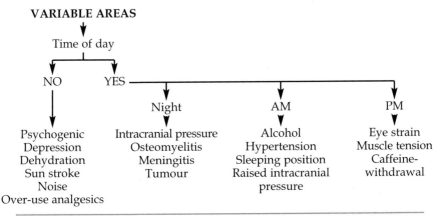

Figure 18.1 Flow chart depicting the different causes of headache.

Causes of symptoms in the head

Bilateral

Hypertension
A vague dull throbbing headache will affect all of the head, especially the occipital region. It is variable, being aggravated by any activity that increases blood pressure.

Cervical
A dull headache or pressure felt in the frontal and occipital areas. If muscle tension irritates the retroauricular nerve, pain is felt behind the ear. The pain is aggravated by neck posture or head movement. If there are spondylotic changes in the neck, it can be associated with dizziness or auditory disturbances.

Eye
The history will link the symptoms with visual effort causing discomfort round the eye or in the temporal areas. There may be an impairment of eye function with reduced visual acuity or increased sensitivity to light.

Unilateral

Trigeminal neuralgia
Mainly affects women between 40-60 years of age. The main complaint is an excruciating spontaneous pain that occurs up to 12 times per day lasting between 30 sec-1 min. The area affected is the sensory distribution of the trigeminal nerve and can be triggered by cold or touch. There may be a slight reddening of the conjunctiva, lacrimation and occasional tingling before the pain starts.

Glossopharyngeal
Mainly affects men between 40-60 years of age. The main symptom is an excruciating spontaneous pain that occurs up to 12 times per day lasting between 30 sec-1 min. The area affected is the retrolingual area to the ear and is triggered by movement or contraction of the pharynx.

Sinus

A dull persistent pressure and pain over the affected sinus. It can be chronic and recurrent or acute related to a nasal infection or reaction to allergy. The pain is aggravated by bending or straining and resolves when the sinus spontaneously drains.

Ear

Infection or increase in pressure within the middle ear causes pain local to the ear. It is more common in children as the eustachian tube is easily blocked. It will resolve with normalisation of the pressure difference by perforation of the eardrum or clearance of the eustachian tube.

Migraine

This affects mainly women between 20-40 years of age. Before the headache begins, there are visual disturbances, nausea, pallor, vomiting, photophobia and fluid retention. The pain builds to an intense throbbing pain in one particular area up to twice a week and can last from a few hours to several days. The exact cause is unknown but hormones, diet, emotion and physical causes have all been implicated.

Cluster

A cluster or histamine headache affects mainly men between 40-60 years of age. The headache is described as an intense, sharp, stabbing and burning pain that occurs between 1-4 times per day lasting from a few minutes to hours particularly over one eye. Attacks are often at night when levels of serotonin or histamine are low. The pain will disturb sleep patterns and can cause personality changes, ipsilateral sweating, lacrimation and either nasal congestion or discharge.

Chapter 19

Chest pain

When a patient presents complaining of chest pain, it is prudent to assume a pathological condition is present and attempts must be made to rule this out during the case history process. Once an initial diagnosis has been reached, a decision must be made as to whether this condition constitutes a red flag to further evaluation. As mentioned in Chapter 1, the red flag may be total, requiring immediate referral to hospital or a general practitioner, or partial, allowing the examination process to continue with a referral if necessary to the patient's general practitioner in the near future.

Causes of chest pain

In most cases the patient will complain of chest symptoms that appear to originate from four specific areas of the chest:-

1. Retrosternal.
2. Central to back.
3. The chest wall.
4. The whole of the chest.

Retrosternal pain: gastrointestinal system

Oesophagitis or hiatus hernia
These can mimic angina but are aggravated by eating or drinking, straining, bending or lying flat, especially within hours of eating a meal. Antacids can help.

Oesophageal spasm
The patient feels solid food becomes stuck in the oesophagus when eating. It can be caused by constriction of the oesophagus or a pouch.

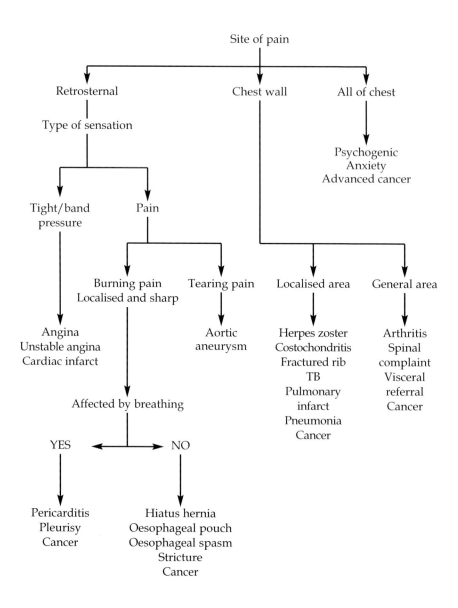

Figure 19.1 Flow chart depicting the different causes of symptoms.

Retrosternal pain: cardiovascular system

Myocardial ischaemia [angina]
Initially retrosternal pain, but can refer to either left or right side of jaw, neck and arm slowly building to a choking/constricting pain. Pain is aggravated by exertion, cold, emotion and stress, and relieved by medication or rest. If unstable, the pattern of pain is less responsive to rest or medication.

Myocardial infarction
Pain radiates to the shoulder, arm, back and jaw. There is a sudden onset of pressure or a tight band with shortness of breath that persists with rest, vomiting, sweating, anxiety, cough, dizziness.

Pericarditis
Pain radiates to the left or right shoulder. There is pain on inspiration or coughing.

Central to back: cardiovascular system

Aortic aneurysm
There is a sudden onset of severe tearing pain.

Chest wall: respiratory system

Pleurisy
Sharp pain on breathing, an audible pleural rub and a history of lung disease present.

Pneumonia
General ill health and signs of infection are present.

Pulmonary infarction
Sudden onset of pain and breathlessness, with general signs of vascular disease present.

Tuberculosis
Signs of generalised ill health are present.

Chest wall: musculoskeletal system

Rib fracture
A history of trauma or osteoporosis is suspected. Pain radiates around the rib with a specific area of tenderness over the fracture site.

Musculoskeletal referral
Affecting the thoracic spine or rib articulations. There is pain on specific movements, deep breathing or exertion. There are signs of joint involvement.

Costochondritis
There is a history of direct trauma to the costochondral junction of a specific rib. Aggravated by deep breathing, coughing, sneezing, rotation. Rest will ease the pain if back is supported.

Chest wall: neurological system

Herpes zoster
Unilateral pain followed by a rash 3-4 days later. It is confined to a single thoracic spinal dermatome.

All chest

Malignancy
Signs of general ill health and weight loss are present.

Psychogenic
There is no diagnostic pattern to the pain. Symptoms are variable for no apparent reason.

Chapter 20

Abdominal pain

When a patient presents complaining of abdominal pain, it is prudent to assume a pathological condition is present and attempts should be made to rule this out during the case history process. Once an initial diagnosis has been reached, a decision must be made as to whether this condition constitutes a red flag to further evaluation. As mentioned in Chapter 1, the red flag may be total, requiring immediate referral to hospital or a general practitioner, or partial, allowing the examination process to continue with a referral if necessary to the patient's general practitioner in the near future.

In most cases of abdominal pain, the symptoms are vague and not specifically felt over the organ causing symptoms. When the symptoms are very acute, localised and accompanied with sweating, specific tenderness or rigidity of the abdominal wall, referral to the hospital should be immediate.

To reach an initial diagnosis, the relationship between the symptoms and food, changes to bowel habit or stool colour, vomiting, swelling or local tenderness should be determined. Figure 20.1 demonstrates how the symptoms from named conditions relate to these specific relationships.

Causes of abdominal pain

Although abdominal symptoms are vague and general, different areas of the gastrointestinal system tend to refer to specific areas of the abdomen as described in the following pages.

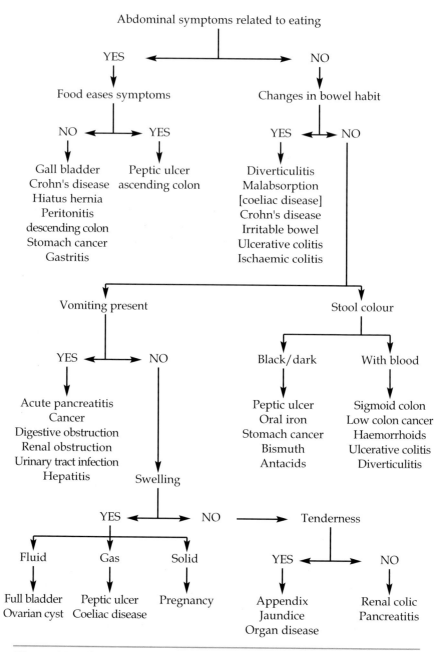

Figure 20.1 Flow chart depicting how symptoms relate to conditions.

Upper abdominal pain: oesophagus and stomach

Oesophagitis or hiatus hernia
Aggravated by eating or drinking, straining, bending or lying flat especially within hours of eating a meal. Antacids can help.

Peptic ulcer
Epigastric pain at predictable times associated with eating food. Antacids help. Can occasionally wake with pain at night.

Gastritis
Epigastric pain occasionally radiates to the left scapula. It may cause dyspepsia, anorexia, nausea, vomiting or melaena. Aspirin or NSAID ingestion can aggravate or cause bleeding.

Upper abdominal pain: hepatic

Gall bladder
Epigastric or right upper abdominal pain to below the right scapula, associated with eating fatty food. When acute, the pain is severe with sweating, pallor and vomiting.

Hepatitis
Right hypochondrium pain on breathing. An audible friction rub can be heard. Liver is palpable below the rib margin.

Central abdominal pain: small intestine and pancreas

Small intestine
Pain several times per minute.

Acute pancreatitis
Epigastric pain occasionally refers to the central back or to the left side. There is severe pain that may be eased by changing position. The chronic form is often found in disease of the biliary tract or in alcoholism.

Crohn's disease
Pain referral depends on the site of the disease process which can affect any part of the digestive system. It is often associated with diarrhoea, weight loss and smoking.

Ulcerative colitis
The pain of the first attack is the most severe, followed by relapses and remissions. It affects only the colon and produces frequent bloody stools. Smoking has no effect.

Malabsorption syndrome
This can affect young adults with non-specific pain that depends on diet. There is weight loss or anaemia and mild abdominal distension.

Lower abdomen: gastrointestinal

Diverticulitis
Pain in the suprapubic area or left iliac fossa with local tenderness and muscular guarding over a palpable mass with associated diarrhoea, rectal bleeding or fever.

Irritable bowel
Colicky or cramping pain with abdominal bloating that increases during the day and is relieved by defecation.

Appendix
Initially the pain is in the central abdomen, radiating to the right iliac fossa.

Coeliac disease
Common in young adults.

Large bowel
There is moderate intermittent pain in the hypogastric or left iliac fossa with several minutes between attacks.

Haemorrhoids
Localised to the site of the anus. There is bleeding and localised pain on pressure or sitting.

Lower abdomen: renal

Renal obstruction
Persistent low grade pain or acute sudden pain between the 12th rib and the iliac crest. Radiates anteriorly to the groin or genitalia and hypochondrium. It is associated with a chill or rigors.

Bladder
Pain in the suprapubic area associated with the desire to urinate.

Urethral
Burning pain localised specifically over the urethra related to urination.

Prostatic
Peroneal pain is rare. There is hesitancy in starting/stopping urination, and frequency and nocturia.

Lower abdomen: gynaecological

Ovarian cyst
Pain in the iliac fossa to the lumbosacral area.

Ectopic pregnancy
There is a sudden excruciating pain over the site of implantation. Possible history of short-term amenorrhoea.

References

Chusid JG. Correlative Neuroanatomy and Functional Neurology, 16th edition. Lange.

Crawford Adams J, Hamblen D. Outline of Orthopaedics, 13th edition. Churchill Livingstone.

Davidson's Principles and Practice of Medicine, 18th edition. Churchill Livingstone.

Goodman CC, Snyder TE. Differential Diagnosis in Physical Therapy, 3rd edition. WB Saunders Co.

Grays Anatomy, 35th edition. Longman.

Hollinshead WH. Textbook of Anatomy, 3rd edition. Harper and Row.

Huskisson EC, Dudley Hart F. Joint Disease: all the arthropathies. John Wright and Sons Ltd.

Kapandji IA. The Physiology of the Joints, volumes 1, 2, 3, 2nd edition. Churchill Livingstone.

Macleod J. Clinical examination, 10th edition. Churchill Livingstone.

Magee DJ. Orthopaedic Physical Assessment, 3rd edition. WB Saunders Co.

McRae R. Clinical Orthopaedic Examination, 3rd edition. Churchill Livingstone.